Psychiatry
and
Religion

*The Convergence of
Mind and Spirit*

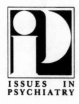

ISSUES IN
PSYCHIATRY

Joseph D. Bloom, M.D., Series Editor

Psychiatry and Religion

*The Convergence of
Mind and Spirit*

EDITED BY

James K. Boehnlein, M.D., M.Sc.

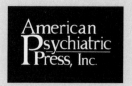

Washington, DC
London, England

Copyright © 2000 American Psychiatric Press, Inc.
ALL RIGHTS RESERVED
Manufactured in the United States of America on acid-free paper
03 02 01   4 3 2
First Edition

American Psychiatric Press, Inc.
1400 K Street, N.W., Washington, DC   20005
www.appi.org

Library of Congress Cataloging-in-Publication Data
Psychiatry and religion / [edited] by James K. Boehnlein. — 1st ed.
    p. cm.   —   (Issues in psychiatry)
    Includes bibliographical references and index.
    ISBN 0-88048-920-0 (alk. paper)
    1. Psychiatry and religion.   I. Series. II. Boehnlein, James K.
    [DNLM: 1. Religion and Psychiatry. 2. Mental Disorders—therapy. 3. Psychiatry.   WM 61 P9735 2000]
    RC455.4.R4   P755   2000
    616.89 21—dc21

                                                                99-040826

British Library Cataloguing in Publication Data
A CIP record is available from the British Library.

To my wife, Mary;
our three children, Katie, Colin, and Kevin;
and my parents, Armand and Betty

Contents

James K. Boehnlein, M.D., M. Sc.

SECTION I

Theoretical Principles and Historical Trends

CHAPTER 1

J. David Kinzie, M.D.

CHAPTER 2

Charles C. Hughes, Ph.D., and
Ronald M. Wintrob, M.D.

CHAPTER 3

W. W. Meissner, S.J., M.D.

CHAPTER 4

Marc Galanter, M.D.

SECTION II

Treatment Issues at the Interface of Psychiatry and Religion

SECTION III

Looking Toward the Future

Contributors

James K. Boehnlein, M.D., M.Sc.
Associate Professor and Director of Medical Student Education in
Psychiatry, Department of Psychiatry, Oregon Health Sciences
University; Associate Director for Education, Mental Illness Research,
Education and Clinical Center (MIRECC), Veterans Affairs Medical
Center, Portland, Oregon

John F. Fergueson, M.Div.
Rector, The Episcopal Church of the Redeemer, Kenmore, Washington

Marc Galanter, M.D.
Professor of Psychiatry and Director, Division of Alcoholism and Drug
Abuse, New York University School of Medicine, New York, New York

Charles C. Hughes, Ph.D.[†]
Professor and Director, Graduate Programs in Public Health,
Department of Family and Preventive Medicine; Professor of
Anthropology, University of Utah, Salt Lake City, Utah

David R. Johnson, M.D., M.P.H.
Assistant Professor of Psychiatry, University of Minnesota, Minneapolis;
Staff Psychiatrist, Veterans Affairs Medical Center, Minneapolis,
Minnesota; Staff Psychiatrist, Center for Victims of Torture,
Minneapolis, Minnesota

J. David Kinzie, M.D.
Professor, Department of Psychiatry, Oregon Health Sciences
University, Portland, Oregon

Harold G. Koenig, M.D., M.H.Sc.
Associate Professor of Psychiatry and Behavioral Sciences; Associate
Professor of Medicine, Center for the Study of Religion, Spirituality, and
Health, Duke University Medical Center and Geriatric Research,
Education, and Clinical Center, Veterans Administration Medical
Center, Durham, North Carolina

[†]Deceased.

David B. Larson, M.D., M.S.P.H.
Adjunct Professor of Psychiatry, Duke University Medical Center, Durham, North Carolina, and Northwestern University Medical School, Chicago, Illinois; President, National Institute for Healthcare Research, Rockville, Maryland

Francis G. Lu, M.D.
Clinical Professor of Psychiatry, University of California, San Francisco; Director, Cultural Competence and Diversity Program, Department of Psychiatry, San Francisco General Hospital, San Francisco, California

Michael E. McCullough, Ph.D.
Director of Research, National Institute for Healthcare Research, Rockville, Maryland

W. W. Meissner, S.J., M.D.
University Professor of Psychoanalysis, Boston College; Training and Supervising Analyst, Boston Psychoanalytic Institute, Boston, Massachusetts

Mary Greenwold Milano, B.A.
Advancement Officer, National Institute for Healthcare Research, Rockville, Maryland

Laurence J. O'Connell, Ph.D., S.T.D.
President and CEO, The Park Ridge Center for the Study of Health, Faith, and Ethics; Adjunct Assistant Professor, Department of Medicine, Stritch School of Medicine, Loyola University, Chicago, Illinois

Landy F. Sparr, M.D., M.A.
Associate Professor of Psychiatry, Oregon Health Sciences University; Acting Chief, Psychiatry Service, Veterans Affairs Medical Center, Portland, Oregon

Andrew J. Weaver, M.Th., Ph.D.
Clinical Psychologist, Department of Psychology, University of Hawaii and Hawaii State Hospital, Honolulu, Hawaii

Joseph Westermeyer, M.D., M.P.H., Ph.D.
Professor of Psychiatry and Adjunct Professor of Anthropology, University of Minnesota; Chief, Psychiatry Service, Veterans Affairs Medical Center, Minneapolis, Minnesota

Ronald M. Wintrob, M.D.
  Clinical Professor of Psychiatry and Human Behavior, Brown University
  School of Medicine, Providence, Rhode Island

Introduction

James K. Boehnlein, M.D., M.Sc.

The ways in which human beings attempt to understand the world, interact with it, and give meaning to their lives have occupied philosophers and scientists for centuries. In the contemporary era, the biological and social sciences and the humanities are frequently in conflict in their attempts to describe the natural world, human behavior, and human conceptualizations of the universe. However, there is also a great deal of convergence among their concepts and constructs that often is obscured because such central elements of human existence inevitably are infused with ideological and political fervor. This book attempts to address both the polarities and the unifying concepts that exist in these domains.

Psychiatry and religion both draw upon rich traditions of human thought and practice. In fact, psychiatry is the branch of medicine that most prominently incorporates the humanities and social sciences in its scientific base and in its treatment of illness. And, in its attempts to explain the full range of human behavior, including behavior associated with mental illness, psychiatry has often needed to go well beyond the world of natural science into the philosophical realm.

In parallel fashion, all religions offer some type of explanation of how the universe was created, how life is maintained, and what happens when life ceases to exist. All religions attempt to give their followers explanations for life's meaning, including rationales for the reality of human suffering. Religious symbols, beliefs, myths, and rites enable individuals and groups to deal with the ultimate conditions of existence that are experienced by members of every society (DeCraemer et al. 1976). From the standpoint of the individual as part of a social unit, religion serves as a source of conceptions of the world, the self, and the relations between them (Geertz 1973). Both religion and psychiatry are concerned with how identity is defined and how this definition is affected by interpersonal and social processes. And, for much of history, the separate functions of religious practice and healing were performed by a single individual in most world cultures. Only with the explosive growth of scientific knowledge in the 20th century have the roles of religious and medical healers become separate.

The major theme of this book, which is reflected throughout its individual chapters, is the proposition that psychiatry and religion are parallel and complementary frames of reference for understanding and describing the human experience and human behavior. Although placing different degrees of emphasis on the relative importance of mind, body, and spirit in defining human nature, the objective and subjective perspectives of psychiatry and religion can be integrated in comprehensive patient care.

A book on psychiatry and religion is particularly timely now because of a resurgence of interest in religious belief and practice in many parts of the world, and because of the increased movement of the world's population, with the subsequent assimilation of a variety of belief systems and practices throughout the world. Mental health providers in developed countries increasingly are treating patients whose backgrounds are much different from their own, so it is important for them to understand cultural belief systems, including religious thought and practice, that relate to mental health and illness.

An increased awareness of religion in contemporary societies has both positive and negative aspects. From a positive point of view, religious belief systems may provide understandable explanations for traumatic life events or provide meaning for individuals or groups. Historically, religious organizations also have funded and operated mental health services in various countries, so it is important for organized psychiatry to be knowledgeable about the historical belief systems and political structures of these organized religions in order to coordinate services and have some influence on their effectiveness.

From a negative point of view, any religious fundamentalism, regardless of belief system, can be damaging not only to individual mental health and social adjustment but also to peaceful coexistence among cultures. Unfortunately, one can look across the globe to Northern Ireland, the Balkans, Africa, and the Middle East for some prominent examples of how the politicalization of religious beliefs can destroy lives and cultures. This, too, is an important area for psychiatry, because survivors of regional war trauma emigrate to other countries, where they subsequently attempt not only to acculturate but also to place their traumatic experiences into a meaningful context.

How a mental health professional defines his or her identity and roles—for example, spouse, parent, colleague, or healer—may also be somewhat influenced by that individual's religious background and beliefs. It is important that practitioners be aware of these factors so that they can maintain proper boundaries between their personal and professional lives. Although psychiatrists, for example, are socialized to their role as healers during long years of medical education and training, their behavior also is influenced by social and cultural values that both precede and coexist with their professional life. Values and ways of thinking can be influenced by family background, peer interaction throughout the life span, and secular and religious education. An awareness of the influence of these diverse factors on identity and professional life is important for the practicing mental health professional. Contemporary decisions in mental health practice require clinicians to place their biomedical knowledge within a social and cultural matrix that has taken centuries to develop.

Therefore, Section I of this volume, consisting of the first four chapters, is concerned with general theoretical principles and historical trends in psychiatry and religion. To explore common roots and to lay a foundation for later chapters, the first chapter by Kinzie provides a cross-cultural perspective by comprehensively describing the history and current status of psychiatry vis-à-vis major world religions. The rich intellectual traditions of Christianity, Judaism, Islam, Hinduism, and Buddhism are compared and contrasted, and their unique contributions to the treatment of the mentally ill are highlighted. During long periods of world history, these religious traditions have made major contributions to how mental illness has been viewed and to the range of treatments patients have received. From our current perspective at the beginning of the 21st century, these contributions can be viewed variably as either regressive or progressive.

In Chapter 2, Hughes and Wintrob define terminology frequently encountered at the interface of religion and psychiatry and explore the extent to which religious healing and rituals have been integrated with medical traditions and healing in a wide variety of cultures throughout history. Specific cultural traditions are highlighted that have interest and relevance to the current multicultural environment in which medicine and psychiatry are practiced.

In Chapter 3, Meissner continues this historical focus by tracing the overlapping concerns of psychoanalysis and religion, including the significant tension between the two domains in the early decades of psychoanalysis. He fully explores the specific cultural traditions and philosophical schools that fueled this early tension. But later in his chapter he highlights features common to both psychoanalysis and religion that can contribute to a truly fruitful dialogue in future years.

Galanter concludes Section I by defining and exploring the phenomenon of cults. Using contemporary examples, he discusses the distinction between cults and religious organizations, describes important characteristics of cults, and highlights psychiatric sequelae of cult involvement.

Section II of this volume is concerned with pragmatic treatment issues at the interface of religion and psychiatry. Extending the cross-cultural perspectives in Section I to the treatment setting, Johnson and Westermeyer in Chapter 5 focus on psychotherapies that either have grown out of religious precepts or have evolved in tandem with religious movements. Psychotherapies that have roots in spiritual and philosophical traditions in both the East and West are described, along with mainstream psychiatric treatments that have incorporated religious concepts or structures.

In Chapter 6, Sparr and Fergueson highlight the importance of including religious and spiritual considerations in comprehensive psychiatric formulations. They specifically focus on the treatment of posttraumatic stress disorder, because the complex existential and spiritual issues associated with trauma and loss are central to both religious faith and the process of posttraumatic recovery. During and after traumatic events, individuals frequently report great cognitive dissonance between what they observe and experience in reality and what they previously believed were stable, secure, and predictable relationships, not only with other individuals but also with the supernatural or the metaphysical. The person recovering from trauma does not have to be religious in a formal sense to experience this dissonance; how the person was socialized to reconcile the pain of loss is what is important (Eisenbruch 1984). Most importantly, including religious and spiritual perspectives in the clinical assessment of patients takes into account the effects of philosophical viewpoints, cultural values, and social attitudes on disease (Fabrega 1975).

What is clinically appropriate in the overlapping roles of mental health practitioners and clergy is continually being debated. In Chapter 7, Larson and colleagues explore this evolving area of mental health practice. Clinicians and clergy share a number of qualities that have been universally identified as central to the efficacy of healers, including communicating the expectation that suffering will be relieved, conveying a knowledgeable manner, drawing together key individuals in the person's life, and generating hope for an improved existence (Frank 1961). In addition, one of the functions of a healer in psychiatric or religious practice is to help reestablish an equilibrium between a person and his or her environment, whether that environment be the natural world, interpersonal relationships, or the person's struggle with meaning, beliefs, or values. Therefore, mental health practitioners and clergy may have separate yet complementary roles in restoring patients to health.

Section III of this volume moves on to a consideration of a number of issues that will affect the future relationship between psychiatry and religion. In Chapter 8, O'Connell explores the complexity of bioethics in a pluralistic society from philosophical and theological perspectives. Religious perspectives are integral to most of the current dilemmas in psychiatric and biomedical ethics, including end-of-life decisions, physician-assisted suicide and euthanasia, abortion, and genetic research. In a multicultural society, the task of developing appropriate ethical guidelines in biomedicine is fraught with great challenges, opportunities, and controversy. Professional ethics cannot be judged in isolation from society's broader ethical traditions, which are influenced by both secular and religious values. With the increasing medicalization of social issues, many physicians are forced to examine their own ethical beliefs. In order to deal with contemporary ethical issues, psychiatrists must be able to draw upon a broadly based intellectual tradition, not only in the biological sciences but also in the humanities and social sciences, which includes the comparative study of religion.

In fact, in the future psychiatrists will increasingly be required to confront numerous ethical and social policy issues with religious components, in addition to meeting patient demands for more comprehensive psychiatric approaches that incorporate spiritual perspectives. In Chapter 9, Lu explores the rationale and purpose of recent mandates for the inclusion of spiritual and religious course content in psychiatric training programs. He describes existing and proposed model curricula that address the knowledge, skills, and attitudes needed by clinicians to sensitively and effectively address religious and spiritual issues in therapy.

In Chapter 10, the final chapter in this volume, Koenig looks to the future to consider how psychiatry and religion can be optimally complementary in meeting the spiritual needs of patients and helping patients in their struggles with suffering, purpose, and meaning. He discusses the role of religious beliefs in mediating human responses to illness and disease and proposes some possible models for integrating science and religion in future psychiatric practice, teaching, and research. The future holds great promise for integrating these concepts in pragmatic ways that will benefit both patients and society.

References

DeCraemer W, Vansina J, Fox RC: Religious movements in central Africa. Comp Stud Soc Hist 18:458–475, 1976

Eisenbruch M: Cross-cultural aspects of bereavement, I: a conceptual framework for comparative analysis. Cult Med Psychiatry 8:283–309, 1984

Fabrega H: The need for an ethnomedical science. Science 189:969–975, 1975

Frank JD: Persuasion and Healing. Baltimore, MD, Johns Hopkins University Press, 1961

Geertz C: The Interpretation of Cultures. New York, Basic Books, 1973

SECTION I

⤴⤸

Theoretical Principles and Historical Trends

⸙ CHAPTER 1 ⸙

The Historical Relationship Between Psychiatry and the Major Religions

J. David Kinzie, M.D.

Religion and psychiatry have had a complicated, sometimes collaborative and sometimes competitive relationship over their long histories. Their relationship is further complicated by the diversity and changes in religion over time, as well as by the evolving medical practice of psychiatry. The major religions are not uniform in their beliefs at the theological level, and each has had to accommodate to local and folk traditions and practices. For example, Christianity encompasses such diverse worship scenarios as High Mass at St. Peter's and an inner-city Evangelical faith healing service. Our understanding of mental illness has also changed greatly over time. Thus, the relationship of psychiatry and religion involves complex belief systems, each diverse and changing. The mentally ill have been with us from the beginning of recorded history, and how they are understood and cared for has often been influenced by the major religions.

Religions affect the care of the mentally ill directly by prescribing treat-

The author greatly appreciates the helpful suggestions given by Crystal Riley, M.A., Tom Kinzie, M.Div., Wen-Shing Tseng, M.D., Larry Sacks, M.D., Dr. Harith Ghassany, and Professor Ala' Aldin Al-Hussaini.

3

ment, such as exorcism for spirit possession, or more broadly by influencing cultures and values, thereby influencing the medical practices of physicians. In this chapter I examine physicians' practices under the various religions. For the purposes of this review, the definition of mental illness will include marked changes in behavior, usually psychosis, but will not include the more nebulous area of general psychological functioning or mental health. Part I provides a historical review of the world's major religions and their influences on the treatment of the mentally ill. Two other areas will be examined if the topic religion has specific teachings about them: alcohol abuse and suicide. Part II surveys the impact of these religions on psychiatric practice in the 20th century.

I begin with a few comments about my own perspectives. As a Western-trained physician, I believe that the rational, clinical scientific approach offers the best perspective on understanding and treating the mentally ill. I also am committed to medical ethics and values that are of primary concern to the physician; for example, the compassionate and humane care of those with mental illness. At their best, religious values inspire humankind to seek ideological and transcendental truths and offer understanding for living. Religions deserve to be taken seriously, but they also need to be held accountable when their high goals are not met. In my professional career, I have worked in a number of cross-cultural settings and have treated patients from all of the major religions discussed in this chapter. I have learned from these patients as well as from colleagues, whose private faiths have included most of the religions described here.

In approaching this topic, I will first provide a historical review of the religion, citing references to mental illness from the religious and medical writings of the period. Reference will be made both to formal religious concepts and practices and to coexisting folk beliefs and customs, with consideration given to how each promoted or detracted from the treatment of psychiatrically impaired individuals. Mention will also be made of alcohol abuse and suicide, because these are topics some religions consider as moral and/or religious issues.

Part I: Historical Impact of the Major Religions on Treatment of Mental Illness

Hinduism

The Hindu religion has a long history of development and is tied to the metaphysical concepts of Indian mythology. During the pre-Vedic period (prior to

1500 B.C.E.), religion was dominated by animistic beliefs, and an extensive world of demons and evil spirits was thought to cause illness (Rao 1975). The Vedic period (1500 to 500 B.C.E.) was named for the four Vedas books, some of which dealt with the prayer incantations and charms for fighting evil spirits thought to cause disease. During the post-Vedic period (600 B.C.E. to 1000 C.E.), a new religion, Hinduism, began to address the needs of human-kind to take charge of its own destiny and to decrease the importance of the gods. These needs were addressed in treatises referred to as *Upanishads*. Because Hinduism eschews systems, it cannot be briefly described. However, a key concept will be mentioned. A sacred power called *Brahman* was the inner meaning of all existence, and the Upanishads encouraged people to cultivate a sense of Brahman, sometimes called *Atman*, in all things and within people. This divine power, Brahman/Atman, prevailed and sustained life (Armstrong 1993).

During this Upanishadic period, Indian medicine began developing a scientific basis. The great physician Caraka lived between the first and second century C.E. He devoted some writings to descriptions of insanity. Caraka's classification of insanity included an endogenous group of disorders produced by imbalances in bodily and mental fluids—humors—and an exogenous group that could be caused by divine punishment, human actions, or failure to fulfill one's duties in a previous life. Recommended treatment ranged from "words of sympathy" to such drastic measures as terrorizing patients with snakes whose fangs had been removed or with threats of immediate execution. Caraka's writings mention no asylums or legal provisions for the care of the mentally ill (Rao 1975).

According to orthodox Hinduism, although humans may desire the acquisition of wealth or sensual pleasures, these cannot really satisfy them; instead, they need to tap the infinite power, Brahman/Atman (this description is taken extensively from Smith 1991). This power may be actualized by yoga, a method of training to help unify internal power. The yoga's pathway may be through reflection, love, work, or psychophysical exercises known in the West as meditation. Hinduism describes various stages of human life, such as student years, marriage, retirement, and eventually renunciation of the world—a time for self-discovery. Hindus further trace an individual's journey through the migration of the body (reincarnation). A person's present life is a product of what he or she has done and wanted in the past—that is, Karma. Because Karma dictates that every action has inexorable consequences, Hindus are committed to moral responsibility.

Two aspects of Hinduism are particularly relevant to this discussion. The first is the importance of symbols, myths, and multiple images of God, which represent the invisible world, a world that cannot be perceived. However, these multiple images imply idolatry and polytheism, a cosmology that may be more prominent at times of illness or disease. Such beliefs are still present in India (Rao 1975). A second aspect of interest is the caste system, which includes the historical stations of life. The castes themselves were ranked hierarchically, but it was assumed through multiple reincarnation that all souls would migrate through all the castes (Smith 1991). The result is, however, exclusivity, rigidity, and severe social discrimination. This was most noticeable among the outcasts, the untouchables at the lowest end of the system. Behavioral expectations for each level of the caste system were not equal, however. The lower caste had less-exacting prohibitions against eating meat or consuming alcohol, a fact that may relate to the development of alcoholism in some Indians.

The emphasis of Hinduism has not been primarily in psychology, but in the existential. Nevertheless, Hindu writings contain information on states of consciousness, peak experiences, and developmental levels. Consciousness, identity, and motivation are addressed in the writings of Hinduism, some of which are similar to Western writings. However, very little is written about severe psychopathology, psychosis, or neurosis. In the 19th century, attempts were made to segregate the mentally ill in India. Stables, barracks, and prisons were used to retain patients. In 1922, these "lunatic asylums" began to be called mental hospitals (Rao 1975).

In the early Vedic period, suicide was sanctioned as a religious ritual, but later, during the Upanishadic period, suicide was condemned. However, suicide was permitted by religious leaders for certain individuals; for example, those suffering from an incurable illness, ascetics, and widows who choose to be cremated with their husbands (i.e., suttee). Most of these practices have disappeared in modern times, but fasting, which can result in suicide by starvation, is still employed, often as a political stratagem.

Buddhism

Buddhism began with Siddhartha Gautama, born in 563 B.C.E. to the son of a ruler of a small kingdom in Nepal (a recent biography of Buddha has been written by Thich Nhat Hanh [1991]). Despite his wealth, he became aware of pain, suffering, and death, and at the age of 29 years he began searching for truth. The path for truth lasted 6 years and led to his Great Awakening. Gautama became Buddha, meaning "to awake and to know." During his 45-year ministry, he founded an order of monks, engaged in public preaching, provided counseling, and challenged contemporary Hindu society for its excessive focus on what he believed were meaningless rituals and traditions. Buddha himself taught a religion devoid of authority, ritual, speculation, and the supernatural. He was empirical, pragmatic, therapeutic, psychological, and egalitarian and appealed to individuals. In many ways, his teachings, as opposed to Buddhism as a religion, have struck a responsive chord in contemporary Western people (Smith 1991).

Buddha's first teachings, the Four Noble Truths, can be briefly summarized as follows: 1) life is suffering, 2) the cause of suffering is desire for private fulfillment, 3) suffering can be relieved by release from narrow self-interest, and 4) the method for this release is through the Eightfold Path. The Eightfold Path involves the right knowledge, speech, behavior, effort, and mindfulness toward others (see Chapter 5 in this volume for a more detailed description). A basic concept of Buddhism denies a personal God, but Nirvana is described as permanent, ageless, deathless, bliss, unborn, a real truth, supreme reality, eternal, and seems to describe the theological term *Godhead*.

Historically, Buddhism separated into two major forms: 1) *Mahayana* ("the big raft"), referring to Buddhism for the people, and 2) *Theravada* ("the way of the elders"), also known as *Hinayana* ("little raft"). The split was over a fundamental issue. For Theravada, Buddha's program is up to the individual; humanity is on its own, as no gods exist. The primary goal of enlightenment is wisdom, and the monastic order *(sangha)* is the heart of the spiritual quest. This form of Buddhism permeates the entire society in Sri Lanka, Burma, Thailand, and Cambodia. For Mahayana, religion incorporates a strong belief in divine powers in which Buddha is a Savior, has elaborate metaphysics and rituals, and emphasizes compassion and life in the world. This form went to China, Korea, Japan, and Tibet. The Japanese form in the West is known as *Zen*.

Mahayana Buddhism reached China around 65 C.E. With its concepts of Indian medicine and demonic theory, this form of Buddhism was compatible with Chinese folk medicine and Taoism (Unschuld 1985). Although many Buddhist ideas were in conflict with the Confucian values that dominated formal medical practice, the Buddhist emphasis on compassion resulted in lasting welfare regulations, and a Buddhist prince founded the first Chinese hospital in the fifth century C.E. (Unschuld 1979). The primary medical influence of Buddhism in China was religious; for example, people prayed to a Chinese Buddhist goddess, Kuan-yen, for relief of suffering. Sometimes Buddhist incantations were added to the prayers. The scientific approaches of Indian medicine never took hold in China, possibly because Buddhism's tolerance, although oriented toward the relief of suffering, was not committed to specific methods or practices (Unschuld 1985). Buddhism's influence contributed to the popular idea of a vast spiritual world that influenced disease (Veith 1975). For example, in Japan, ghosts of departed dissolute priests could become emissaries of the devil and drive people to madness. Because the mental illness was the result of demonic possession, the patient was considered to be beyond the help of medical care, and treatment was then in the hands of the priests. Since individuals were not personally responsible for their mental illness, the mentally ill were not subject to personal attacks or scorn (Veith 1975).

Formal Buddhist writing includes few comments on psychosis (Walsh 1988), even though Zen monasteries often became temporary refuges for psychotic patients. However, a specific method of treatment developed in Japan for neurosis, Morita therapy, was patterned after Zen Buddhism. In Morita therapy, similar to a Zen ritual, patients undergo complete bed rest, isolation for a week, then a period of work in a garden, and finally reintegration into society. Instead of catharsis or even discussion of the patient's subjective life, there is a ritualized reeducation to free the patient from self-absorption and egocentricity (Veith 1975). (Morita therapy is described in more detail in Chapter 5 of this volume.)

Confucianism and Taoism

Confucianism and Taoism are discussed here together, as they influenced Chinese medicine during the same time span, albeit in very different ways.

Confucius (K'ung-Fu-tzu) known as the First Teacher, brought some basic values of Chinese culture to a focus, and his influence has lasted to the current time. Chinese do not regard Confucianism as a religion (W. S. Tseng, personal communication, October 1995), but it is considered a religion by others and has had a major influence on Chinese thought and ethics. Born in 551 B.C.E., he failed in his life's goal of politics but became a great teacher. His style was informal and democratic and his teaching method was Socratic. Confucius lived at a time of constant warfare, and the appeal of his message was the maintenance of social cohesion through a statement of deliberate tradition of proper social relationships. For Confucius, social life involved mature people with self-affirming largesse of heart who live with propriety. Confucianism places great emphasis on five key relationships: parent and child, husband and wife, older siblings and junior siblings, older friend and junior friend, and ruler and subject. Three of these relationships involve the family, an important Chinese institution, and three focus on looking up to one's elders or superiors. Confucianism also asserts that the top "partner" in these relationships must be correct—that is, the ruler seeks the welfare of his underlings as his first concern. Confucius attended to proper conduct in the moral order and changed the emphasis from the spirit world to the living world, ancestor worship to filial piety (Smith 1991; Tseng 1973b). Confucianism became the basic instruction for government officials from 130 B.C.E., until the collapse of the empire in 1905. Confucianism became, in effect, the state religion. Its impact in China and East Asia on restraint and subtlety in social relationships cannot be overemphasized.

Taoism originated with Lao-tzu, born 604 B.C.E., of whom very little is known. Whether he even actually lived is a mystery. Lao-tzu is credited with writing the *Tao Te Ching* ("The Way and Its Power"), the basic Tao text. This work probably did not exist in its present form until the third century B.C.E. *Tao*, a key concept, refers to the Way of ultimate reality of the universe and of human life. Tao as a concept probably antedates Lao-tzu and is common to all Chinese (Veith 1949). Tao also refers to power. In this sense, Taoism has a philosophical branch and a religious branch. Philosophical Taoism is not so much a movement as an attitude toward life and search for knowledge. Religious Taoism took form in the second century and promoted a multitude of deities and sacred texts. A succession of religious Taoist leaders continues in Taiwan. Like philosophical Taoism, religious Taoism tries to maximize the power of Tao but often with magical and occult techniques. Taoism in all its forms stands on several values important in Chinese life: humility, the rejection of self-assertiveness and competition, attunement toward nature, simplicity in thought and action, and, most notably, the tolerance of opposites as pictured in the classic Yin–Yang symbol. Yin–Yang summarizes life's opposites: male–female, hot–cold, light–dark, positive–negative. These opposites really are phases in the wholeness of life.

The main emphases of Chinese religions seem to balance each other. Confucianism is formal, rational, socially responsible, and emphasizes human affairs. Taoism is mystical and romantic, encourages spontaneity and naturalness, and searches for that which is beyond human affairs.

The development of Chinese medicine, and especially psychiatry, is long and complex. Medicine was separated from sorcery in the Pre-Chou period (2800 to 220 B.C.E.) (Tseng 1973a). During the Chou period, medical writings were based on more clinical experience than the natural philosophy of the Pre-Chou period, but basic knowledge of anatomy and physiology was still lacking. The scholarly Confucian view was that disease, and particularly madness, was due to a violation of some social order, an imbalance of Yin and Yang, or an infringement on Tao (Veith 1975).

Insanity was recognized as a disease in the oldest Chinese text, *The Yellow*

Emperor's Classic of Internal Medicine (Huang Di Nei Ching Su Wen), probably completed in the early Han dynasty (206 B.C.E.–25 C.E.). This book describes harmful, evil disturbances affecting Yin and Yang that cause wildness, insanity, loss of speech, and anger (Veith 1949). The great Chinese physician Chang Chung-Ching (150–210 C.E.) wrote a medical text, *Shang Han Lun*. The text has less of a suggestion of the supernatural elements of disease and no suggestion that diseases are punishment for actions (Epler 1988; Hsu and Peacher 1981). Another text by Chang Chung-Ching described several treatments for mania and irrational behavior (Su-Yen and Hsu 1983).

China has a long folk history of demonic traditions in medicine in which a variety of deities were believed to influence health and disease (Unschuld 1985; Veith 1975). As a result of Tao and Buddhist influence, supernatural influences were found in the formal medical writing again, although it disappeared by the Sung dynasty (960 C.E.). It has been suggested that the Confucian scholars attempted to maintain control over medical practices, especially over independent Tao and Buddhist practitioners (Unschuld 1979).

Chinese medicine never really defined a dichotomy between mind and body. Emotions were known to affect body organs and vice versa. Medicines and acupuncture could reduce the Yin–Yang imbalance. However, demonic concepts continued to exist in medical texts until the 19th century, and treatments were often undertaken by Taoist priests. Other writers thought demons only attacked those whose lives were not correct in the Confucian sense. In the early 1900s, a physician described the treatment for evil possession involving amulets and incantation (Unschuld 1985).

Despite the demonic concepts of mental illness, there were no social attacks on the mentally ill, and generally, they were well tolerated. The Confucian concept of correct family relationships also gave protection for ill family members, whether they were elders with senile dementia or the mentally ill young. Suicide, traditionally, has been rare in Chinese society, as it is an affront to ancestral devotion (Veith 1975).

Judaism

Judaism has had a profound impact on Western culture and, specifically, Western medicine (Armstrong 1993; Smith 1991). Yahweh, the Jewish God, evolved from a personal and tribal deity to the ultimate and only God (Miles 1995). Monotheism was one of the major achievements of Judaism. God was believed to be passionate and very involved in human affairs, in striking contrast to the remote and fickle gods of the Greeks. God was good and righteous, and His creations—the world and its people—were good. This resulted in a belief in the importance of material aspects of life, and hence the emphasis on social services and humanitarian activities. Jews found meaning in their history, with its relationship to God's intervention in their lives, and a strong moral code as illustrated by the Ten Commandments. Justice was also a basic Jewish value, reinforced by the remarkable prophets, Amos, Hosea, Micah, Jeremiah, and Isaiah, who challenged corruption in the social order before the first fall of Jerusalem. From the time of captivity in Babylon following the destruction of Jerusalem in 586 B.C.E., the Jews struggled with the meaning of suffering and the importance of their covenant with God.

Jews never propagated an official creed but placed more emphasis on practices and traditions that are rooted in sharing life with God. The basic manual for respecting and honoring life is the Torah, the first five books of the Bible. The Mosaic law and its oral traditions were brought up to date by Jewish scholars in a series of treatises called the Talmud, first compiled in the fourth century. In the earliest passages of the Talmud the Rabbis described God as a mystical phenomenon. The Rabbis thought that God did not want people to suffer and that the human body was to be honored and cared for.

Judaism has had a long relationship with medicine. One of the earliest statements was by Maimonides, the 12th-century rabbi–physician who promoted good physical health as a means of serving God. The ethical imperative to heal also has its roots in Leviticus, Deuteronomy, and the Talmud by the multiple injunctions to imitate God by healing the sick. Mental health is as important as physical health, according to Maimonides' writings in the 13th century (Feldman 1986).

Early references to mental illness appear in the Bible. Deuteronomy 6:5 reads, "The Lord will strike you with madness," implying that insanity could be caused by divine punishment. The depression and probable suicide of Israel's King Saul are described in Samuel 31:4, and Daniel 4:29–30 recounts the strange psychosis of Nebuchadnezzar, the ruler of Babylon, who lived in 605–562 B.C.E. (Alexander and Selesnick 1966).

The Jewish concern with humanitarian aspects of medicine and psychiatry has a long history. As early as 490 C.E., there was a hospital in Jerusalem solely for the mentally ill (Alexander and Selesnick 1966). Jewish physicians made early contributions to psychiatry, including Asaph in the sixth or seventh century and Donnolo in the 10th century (Miller 1975). Both were dependent on the humoral theories of Hippocrates and Galen but rejected magical causes of illness. Maimonides, in the 12th century, made contributions to medicine by describing the anatomy of the brain and psychiatric disorders. He subscribed to the Jewish concept of prevention rather than treatment, because if one is ill one cannot serve the Lord properly (Rosner 1996). In his recognition of the influence of emotions on bodily function, he is considered the father of psychosomatic medicine. This flowering of Jewish medicine was followed by a prolonged period of folk medicine that treated mentally ill patients as if they were controlled by spirits and devils (Miller 1975). In 1730, Hasidism, a Jewish charismatic religion, was founded by Israel Ben Eliezer, a faith healer, who healed the sick with herbal remedies, amulets, and exorcism (Armstrong 1993). Sigmund Freud and the psychoanalytic movement has had a large influence on 20th-century Western psychiatry. Freud's inner circle included Sándor Ferenczi, Karl Abraham, Max Eitingon, Otto Rank, Hanns Sachs, and only one non-Jew, Ernst Jones. Jones has commented on the effect of Freud's Jewishness on his attitudes and ideas. Freud's firmness in holding on to his ideas is attributed to the capacity of Jews to stand their ground in the face of opposition (Miller 1975).

In addition to Saul's suicide, there are frequent mentions of suicide in the Bible and in ancient Jewish writings in the Talmud (Rosner 1972). Generally, Judaism regards suicide as a criminal act—a denial of God's divine creation of man—and it is forbidden by Jewish law. However, suicide is permitted under a few special circumstances, such as martyrdom for a religious cause. The strict definition of suicide (i.e., suicide as a criminal act), however, does not apply to suicide by children, by those under severe emotional and physical stress, and by those not in full possession of their faculties. Mentally ill individuals who commit suicide may be accorded full burial honors.

Christianity

Christianity began with the Jewish carpenter, Jesus, born in Palestine around 4 B.C.E. He had a teaching and healing ministry lasting between 1½ and 3 years and was executed at the age of 33. Jesus was a charismatic worker of wonders in a long Jewish tradition and was preceded by John the Baptist. He stressed Yahweh's compassion, and he preached to all members of society across social barriers. He went against the social grain and opposed the holiness codes of the Jewish authorities, which he felt created social division. The Jesus of history evolved, through his followers, to the Christ who had become God in human form, and thus an elaborate theology was produced. Jesus' teachings are parallel to the Old Testament and the Talmud but are fresh and vivid, with an appeal to human imagination. (For a more recent view of what Jesus said according to some current scholars, see Funk and Hoover 1993.) In simple language, he taught of God's love, and his life is described as extraordinary; people believed that they had seen God in human form.

The Christian church, however, came from a faith in Jesus' resurrection and that he continued to live. The early church believed in Jesus Christ, the Son of God, who transformed the lives of believers, Jews and Gentiles, by their feeling that in some way the resurrected Christ was with them and, as a group (church), they were part of Christ's body. The theology of the church, begun by the apostle Paul and developed by the church fathers over several centuries, hinged on a few key concepts: incarnation, how God became human; atonement, God's relieving humankind from sin; and the Trinity, the concept of God being three in one. The need for atonement, especially from original sin of sexuality described by Saint Augustine, implied that a chronically flawed humanity was alienated from itself, and particularly men were alienated because of the tempting seductiveness of women (Armstrong 1993). This belief was to have later consequences for psychiatry. A related Christian development was the concept of Satan, whose demonic influence was attributed to Jews, Romans, Gentiles, and even dissident Christians, including a variety of heretical groups (Pagels 1995). Around 180 C.E., Bishop Irenaeus contributed to the construction of orthodox Christianity by claiming sole access to church doctrines against all heretics. The contradiction and tension within Christianity between those who prayed for reconciliation alongside those who opposed them, and those who taught and acted that "heretical" enemies were evil and beyond redemption, has been with the church much of its history.

Healing and exorcism played a central role in Jesus' ministry, according to the Gospel writers. These miracles often were portrayed not as ends in themselves, but as a sign of Jesus' messianic credentials (Ferngren 1992). Other New Testament records indicate some healing by ordinary means, but there also were reports of others who were not healed. Not until the fourth or fifth century did anointing the sick become a common Christian practice. Indeed, in the second century, Christian healing seemed to be minimal compared with that attributed to Asclepius, the Greek god of healing. According to early Christian writers, the third century saw a rise in supernatural healing and exorcism. This was also seen in Jewish and pagan circles, and reflected a growing belief in the demonic etiology of disease. In the fourth century, Christianity became a religion of healing through the laying on of hands, prayer, fasting, the invocation of Christ's name, the sign of the cross, and exorcism. The care of the sick became a prominent emphasis of the early church and an expected duty of deacons and deaconesses. This revolutionized the attitude toward the sick. The Christian community offered extended, organized community care to themselves and to others as well. This was Christianity's unique contribution to medical care. The development of "hospitals" in the late Roman Empire offers an example of continuity in medical traditions, from the classic Greek to Eastern Christendom. It was in the Eastern church that Jesus was often described as the great physician (Allan 1990). In the Near East, Christians developed and maintained a monopoly on the medical profession, which extended into the Islamic period.

During the European Middle Ages, the understanding of mental health was dominated by witchcraft, demonology, and possession. Sin was considered the cause of illness, and especially mental illness, and psychiatry consisted of predominantly prescientific demonology (Alexander and Selesnick 1966; Zilboorg 1941). The belief in magic by the common people and the work of the devil (witchcraft) became joined, and it became the duty of the church to attack these evils (Bromberg 1975). The enlightened view of the Franciscan monk Bartholomew, who advocated a reasonably restrained treatment of the mentally ill, was seen as an exception (Bromberg 1975). These views have been subjected to critical review. In a study of pre-Crusades chronicles, only 16% of mental illness cases described were attributed to sin or wrongdoing (Knoll and Bachrach 1984). During the same period, only 21% of cases of physical disease were attributed to sin (Knoll and Bachrach 1986). Medieval sources indicate that mundane proximal causes, humoral imbalance and intemperate diet, overwork, and greed were commonly used to explain illnesses. A review of the 17th-century practice of an astrologer/healer in England indicated that about 25% of individuals suffering from mental illness believed that the disorder was caused by witchcraft or harmful spirits, a concept that was more inclusive than sin alone (MacDonald 1981).

Although controversy exists regarding the influence of witchcraft and sin in causing disease during the Middle Ages, there is little doubt that the publication of *Malleus Maleficarum (the Witches' Hammer)* by two Dominican monks, James Sprenger and Heinrich Kraemer, 1487, led to severe cruelty toward the mentally ill. The book describes the existence of witches and devils and how to identify them. A central idea throughout the book was that women were closely identified with sin and the devil: "all witchcraft comes from carnal love which is in women insatiable" (Zilboorg 1935, p. 56). The fusion of witchcraft, insanity, and heresy gave the church authority to act. As a result of this authority and the resultant Inquisition, many witches were identified and probably many thousands of mentally ill were burned at the stake or tortured to death. The last witch was decapitated in Switzerland in 1782 (Zilboorg 1941). Unique in medieval Christianity was the religious and theological justification of cruelty toward the mentally ill.

Nevertheless, there were voices of reason and humanism during that time. The most thoughtful was a Christian physician, Johan Weyer (1515–1588), whom Zilboorg (1935, 1941) has called the first psychiatrist. Weyer looked at patients as they were, people whose psychological characteristics were to be understood as natural phenomena. He spent much of his professional life devoted to objective description of the mentally ill. His work systematically refuted the basis for *Malleus Maleficarum,* although he himself probably believed in devils.

Christian hospitals, even in the Middle Ages, kept the tradition of kindness and humane treatment, including that for the mentally ill. In 1311, monastic care was established by the Knights of St. John on the Island of Rhodes. Other hospitals were established along a route to the Holy Land in France, Switzerland, and Italy during the 11th, 12th, and 13th centuries (Bromberg 1975). Monasteries assumed the burden of care for the feeble-minded and for psychotic patients. One of the first hospitals exclusively for the mentally ill was founded in Gheel, Belgium, in the 13th century. In the Valcenic Asylum (founded in 1409), patients were treated with kindness. There is evidence of humanizing treatment of the mentally ill in Italy in the 15th century, and in France around 1530 under the influence of the reformist Vipes. The celebrated removal of the chains of the mentally ill by Philippe Pinel in France occurred in 1793, which began the era of moral treatment. In America, Quakers William and Henry Tuke were horrified by the terrible conditions of patients in asylums and started the York Retreat. York Retreat became a reflection of the Society of Friends' practical mysticism and the concept of closeness to God through the unity of humankind (Bromberg 1975).

The age of enlightenment and the moral treatment of the mentally ill continued in an uneven manner in the 18th and 19th centuries in Europe and America. The improvements occurred more because of general concepts of humanism and the medicalization of the care of the mentally ill rather than by direct religious influence. The role of Christianity in psychiatric treatment became even less central in the 20th century. With the advent of psychotherapies and counseling techniques, and later the development of Christian counseling, religious concepts were merged with psychotherapeutic approaches (see Chapter 5 in this volume).

Islam

The prophet Mohammed was born into the leading tribe of Mecca in Koreish (Quraysh) in 570 C.E. After 15 years of preparation, including solitude and all-night vigils, he came to believe that Allah, the high God of the Arabic pantheon, was the one and only God, the same God worshiped by Jews and

Christians. Allah as the true and only God had been confused with other Arabic gods because of the corruption of monotheism by polytheistic beliefs of the time. After this revelation around 610, Mohammed received his commission as "the anointed one" following the prophets Abraham, Moses, and Jesus. Then began a life given to God and humanity, despite persecution and opposition to his ministry. In 622, he escaped Mecca and made a migration (in Arabic *Hijra*) to Medinese. That event became a turning point for Muslims and the start of their calendar. In Medina, Mohammed became a skillful politician and statesman. He led an unpretentious life, and as an administrator was known for his justice and mercy. The Medinese eventually were able to capture Mecca, and Mohammed returned as the conqueror. A mass conversion to the Muslim faith subsequently occurred. When Mohammed died in 632, most of Arabia was under his control. He was a man of exceptional genius and he had united the tribes of Arabia with a unique form of spirituality that suited their cultural traditions. In the next 70 years, Islam spread to most of the Middle East, North Africa, and Spain (Smith 1991).

Mohammed regarded that God had performed only one miracle through him—the Koran itself (*al-qur'an* in Arabic). The words of the Koran came to Mohammed over a period of 23 years. The Koran is divided into 114 chapters, or *surahs*, whose main purpose is to proclaim God's omnipotence and mercy and man's total dependence on Him. In the Koran, God speaks in the first person, and Muslims tend to view each word or sentence as His separate revelation (Smith 1991).

The first of the Five Pillars of Islam is the simple affirmation and creed, "There is no God but God and Mohammed is the prophet." The second pillar is prayer; its frequency is fixed at five times per day. The third pillar is charity. The fourth pillar, fasting, is required during Ramadan, the fasting month—the holy month commemorating when Mohammed received his revelation and 10 years later made his historic migration from Mecca to Medina. To observe Ramadan, Muslims are not to eat or drink from sunup to sundown. The fifth pillar, pilgrimage, is prescribed for those who can afford to journey to Mecca once during their lifetime.

Islam brought a vast change to the moral and social order of Arabia and established a specific social order in which faith, politics, and society were joined. In the areas of social injustice, special-interest groups, the status of women, race relations, and the conduct of war, Islam made many major advances. Mohammed taught respect for the natural world order, which allowed Muslims to approach science much sooner than the Christians. Muslim sayings and traditions were collected, but not completed, during the Prophet's lifetime. These directives became known as "the medicine of the

Prophet." The Prophet stressed that "for every disease there is a cause," which strongly persuaded followers to seek treatment. He understood psychological factors in disease, as indicated by his saying "He who is overcome by worries, will have a sick body." Muslim theologians believed that the Prophet advocated combining medicine with divine healing and physical treatment with psychological treatment (Baasher 1975).

The enlightened early Muslim leaders promoted scientific knowledge and assimilated other cultures. The first Muslim hospital was said to have been established in Baghdad between 786 and 809 C.E. and modeled after Christian hospitals, although hospitals based on Indian medicine may have been established earlier. Clearly, there were many Christian physicians in the early Islamic period, and they had great influence in the introduction of Greek medicine. The earliest provisions for the mentally ill were in a hospital in what is now Cairo, in 872–873 (Dols 1987a), and wards for the mentally ill were invariably found in Islamic hospitals (Dols 1987b). Descriptions of treatment at the hospitals indicate that conditions were quite harsh but that doctors seemed interested in the patients and used a variety of therapeutic techniques. In Moorish Spain, the asylums in Zaragoza, Granada, and Barcelona, influenced by Islamic tradition, were described as humanistic institutions (Bromberg 1975).

Although Islam forbade dissections of the human body, the absence of a demonic theory of disease among its tenets allowed advancements in medical knowledge and practice. Medical curricula included the Greek works of Galen; in fact, an interesting case report exists in which a Medieval Arabian physician employed psychotherapy techniques similar to those of Galen (Hajal 1983). By the ninth century, medical textbooks were being written by Muslim physicians. The Arabic medical profession was cosmopolitan and sophisticated, open to members of all faiths. Nonetheless, nonprofessional charlatans did thrive (Leiser 1983).

The illustrious Arab physician Rhazes (865–926) was a brilliant clinician who gave excellent descriptions of illnesses, including mental ones. Apparently he used psychotherapy in a primitive but dynamic way (Baasher 1975). Avicenna (980–1037), the most brilliant of Arab physicians, wrote *The Canon Medicine*, which was used as the medical bible until the 16th century. His excellent clinical descriptions (albeit accompanied by some medical misinformation) included astute observations on psychosomatic medicine (Baasher 1975). The 11th-century physician Ibn Jazlah described melancholia with delusions, manic depression, and psychosis, although he attributed these disorders to humors (Graziani 1980).

Sufism, the mystic form of Islam that stresses an inner message and the desire to encounter God directly in one's lifetime, originally gathered around spiritual masters. Sufism emphasized that health and illness depended on God alone. As it grew in popularity in the 12th century, Sufism created marked tension between some Muslims and the medical profession. The Sufi were, in turn, criticized by orthodox Muslim theologians for their views, including their rejection of medicine (Dols 1984).

The Koran is precise about suicide: "Do not kill yourself, for God was merciful to you" (Baasher 1975). The prohibition against wine was introduced gradually, and the general rule in Islam became that any drug that clouds the mind is prohibited. Islam strongly opposes homosexuality.

During the Middle Ages, the care of the mentally ill in Islam continued in an intellectual tradition that provided an academic approach unavailable in medieval Europe. A 14th-century hospital in Cairo had a separate ward for psychiatric patients. A number of drugs were produced by Arab scientists; a 13th-century work listed 1,400 drugs. Avicenna used rauwolfia in the treatment of acute mental symptoms.

After the 14th century, magic and superstition began to creep back into the medical works of Muslim writers. Sufi and its mystical path (Tanga) developed religious healing. The emergence of magical religious practice in the Arab world came as the political Muslim states declined during the 14th century.

The influence of European educators in the 19th century caused a major shift in Arab medicine, and the first Western medical school was founded in Cairo in 1876. By the 20th century, psychiatric institutions were developed on the models of European mental hospitals.

Part II: Impact of the Major Religions on 20th-Century Psychiatry

The 20th century has seen a large increase in the interaction of major religions and psychiatry. This interaction usually has occurred not in the treatment of the seriously mentally ill, but more in the treatment of neurosis, psychosomatic diseases, and life's existential issues. A brief survey of some of these interactions follows.

Hinduism

In the Western world, yoga and relaxation techniques are now practiced widely. These techniques are based on some of the psychophysiological methods of Hinduism that attempt to achieve control of bodily functions and to gain peace of mind. Some studies have indicated that such methods may help alleviate anxiety and psychosomatic disorders (Vahia et al. 1966).

Anecdotal accounts from Hindu mythology have been useful in the psychotherapy of rural Indian patients (Shamasundar 1993).

The Tamil Indians worship a Hindu deity known as Lord Murugan, to whom they make vows in times of illness or trouble. During Thaipusam, a festival honoring Murugan, worshipers fulfill their vows by performing rituals in which they enter an analgesic trance and allow their bodies to be pierced by special hooks and needles. This dramatic ceremony has been studied by psychiatrists, who suggest that a central opiate mechanism and the limbic system may be involved in maintaining analgesia (Simons et al. 1988).

Buddhism

The Eastern philosophies, particularity those of Theravada Buddhism, have had an impact on Western psychotherapies. As indicated above, some of the experimental work on the physiology of trance and mediation has made the information more understandable. Even more important, however, is the emphasis on certain values that may have been deficient in Western psychotherapies. The Buddhist focus on existential and transpersonal issues, and details of states of consciousness and peak experiences, seems to be beyond Western psychotherapy (Walsh 1988). Some Buddhist approaches deal with the modern spiritual vacuum not by denying it, but rather by going into the emptiness and by emphasizing direct personal experience (Atwood and Maltin 1991). A specific method of direct experience has been meditation, especially Vipissanna, or insight meditation. Such meditative practices may enhance traditional psychotherapy practices, as has been expertly described by Epstein (1995). However, as more experience has been gained with meditation, contraindications have been appreciated, as in the need to strengthen ego boundaries or work through complex personal dynamics (Bogart 1991). For a spiritually deprived patient, meditation may offer more relief and acceptance than traditional psychotherapies.

The Zen-derived Morita therapy has recently been suggested as a form of treatment for social phobias or specific obsessions, which may promote a higher cure rate than standard treatments (Ishimaru-Tseng 1996). (The Eastern philosophies and their impact on Western psychotherapies are described more fully in Chapter 2 of this volume.)

Judaism

As discussed previously, Freud and his followers, largely Jewish, had a great impact on 20th-century psychiatry. Freud's last work, "Moses and Monotheism" (Freud 1939/1964), is a highly speculative account of the relationship between the Jewish people and Moses, and may reveal Freud's conflicts with his own Jewishness (Young 1992). The field of psychotherapy is replete with individuals of Jewish descent. In one study of psychotherapists in American cities, 52% were found to be Jewish, and Jews tend to be overrepresented in studies of outpatient psychotherapy practices (Sauna 1992). In an extensive review of the literature, Sauna concluded that a higher percentage of Jews than of other ethnic groups seek psychotherapy, particularly that of a psychoanalytical nature. Jews seem to have a higher rate of depression and neurosis and a lower rate of schizophrenia compared with other ethnic groups. The suicide rate is low among Jews, and alcohol and drug use are minimal (Sauna 1992). With the weakening of the relationships to Jewish identity, alcoholism and drug abuse may now be increasing. Clearly, Jews constitute a heterogeneous group (i.e., Judaism comprises Orthodox, Conservative, and Reform divisions) and live in diverse countries and cultures; thus, attempts at generalization can only be tentative. Although American literature tends to depict Jews as particularly prone to guilty feelings, one study has found that guilt is less common among Jewish depressed than among Christian depressed patients (Ball and Clare 1990).

Judaism, and perhaps all religions, have been deeply affected by one of the darkest events of history, the murder of two-thirds of European Jewry during World War II—the Holocaust. As Nozick (1989) has pointed out, some response to this cataclysmic episode is called for; however, what that response should be is not clear, for the whole human family has been stained. The Holocaust represents a problem for Jewish theologians seeking to understand the actions of God. For Christians, the problem may be just as profound. Did Christ, in dying for our sins, past and future, have such a horrible sin in mind—one that even seemed to be chosen by humanity? Is there any redemption left for the human race? The Holocaust and other atrocities of the 20th century raise troubling and possibly unanswerable theological questions for humanity.

For psychiatry, a series of clinical reports have documented the profound long-term effects for survivors of the Holocaust (see review in Kinzie and Goetz 1996). One such survivor, psychiatrist Victor Frankl (1963), has written in a truly remarkable way of his search for meaning from the death camp experience.

Christianity

Reforms of the appalling conditions in mental hospitals started by Christian reformers have now been accomplished in much of the world. Governmental and medical guidelines and economic pressures have greatly improved conditions for mental patients. Indeed, there even may have been the overreaction of discharging people from hospitals before they were able to cope on their own. Psychiatric concepts, including those from psychoanalysis, have become a familiar language to mainstream clergy, who use psychological and counseling techniques. Pastoral counselors are supported by active clinical programs and professional organizations and even have shifted away from parish-based practices. A study of formal counseling activities revealed that clergy constitute a heterogeneous group (Mollica et al. 1986). In the study, mainstream clergy engaged in limited counseling activities but felt comfortable making professional referrals; however, evangelical and black clergy devoted a higher percentage of time to counseling but had very limited access to specialized mental health services. (Pastoral care is discussed more fully in Chapter 7 of this volume.)

There has been rapid growth in Pentecostal and Fundamentalist Christian healing that falls outside the professional pastoral counseling movement. As has been well described by Favazza (1982), such healing has a long history; it has attracted a middle-class following and is sometimes practiced in mainstream Christian churches. Some faith healers employ psychiatric concepts (e.g., the importance of childhood conflicts in causing mental illness) and recognize that healing, even with prayer, may be gradual. However, supernatural explanations such as evil spirits and demonic possession remain prominent, especially among Fundamentalist "hard-liners."

Catholic theology strongly condemns suicide, which may explain the low rates of suicide in Catholic European countries compared with Protestant countries. However, the highest death rates from liver cirrhosis (reflecting alcoholism) are in Catholic countries (Mexico, Chile, Puerto Rico) in the Americas. The reasons for these high rates of alcohol abuse are certainly complex and transcend religious orientation (Desjarlais et al. 1995).

Islam

Reports from parts of the Islamic world indicate that traditional healing practices are still employed, sometimes incorporating readings from the Koran (Al-Issa 1989; Al-Sabair 1989). Modern hospitals with psychiatric units are found in all parts of the Islamic world but are probably available to only a small percentage of the population, given that many Islamic countries are still poorly developed. In some areas, Islamic communities have utilized the mosque as a center for helping the mentally ill. Group meetings held in the mosque help individuals avoid isolation and promote mutual cooperation in the community (Chaudhry 1990). Collaborations of religious leaders and mental health professionals have occurred in Cairo. In Saudi Arabia, group psychotherapy employing elements of Islamic worship has been effective in relieving psychiatric symptoms as well as in regrounding patients in Islamic spiritual faith (Al-Radi and Al-Mahdy 1989).

Islam strictly forbids alcohol use, and alcoholism is described as rare in Saudi Arabia. However, there are suggestions that alcohol use is a growing problem in Algeria (Al-Issa 1989) and in Iran (Roohanna 1986). On the basis of positive blood alcohol levels found in cases of trauma, some investigators have concluded that alcohol abuse may be a significant problem in Kuwait (Bibal and Angelo-Khattan 1988).

Suicide is an unforgivable sin in Islam, and studies have shown a low rate of suicide in Muslim countries (Al-Sabair 1989). Suicide in South Asia is lower in Muslims than in Hindus (quoted in Desjarlais et al. 1995). Recordings of suicide attempts occurring in Jordan have shown a decline during the holy months of Ramadan (Dradkey 1992).

Fundamentalism

There has been a trend since the 1970s in Judaism, Christianity, and Islam toward a rise in religiosity known as "fundamentalism" (Armstrong 1993). These movements are highly political, stress literal and strict adherence to sacred writing, and tend to be intolerant in their outlook. Christian fundamentalists campaign vigorously for their views on certain moral issues (e.g., homosexuality, abortion). Some assert that members of other religions are destined for hell. Muslim fundamentalists have overturned governments, mounted insurrections, plotted assassinations, and threatened death to the enemies of Islam. Jewish fundamentalists have become increasingly militant and in Israel have vowed to drive out Arab inhabitants forcibly, if necessary, and to block peace processes. These religious extremists are using "God" to deny others their human rights and are substituting a primitive ideal of tribal superiority for a God of compassion. Al-Mutlaq (1996) has outlined some of the nonspiritual rewards of Islamic fundamentalism; these include status, safe expression of hostility, and covering up of personal or professional inadequacies. Such mechanisms could similarly be operating for Christian and Jewish fundamentalists.

For those who do not follow the fundamentalist view of proper behavior, whether as a matter of personal conscience or as the result of emotional and mental stress, the condemnation of fundamentalists can be severe. Intolerant attitudes take a heavy toll on those seen as different, especially the mentally ill. It is hoped that the compassion in all religions remains a guiding force that allows humankind to understand and treat those who suffer from mental illness.

Summary and Conclusions

Perhaps more than other areas of medical practice, the study and treatment of mental illness have been influenced by societies' views of the spiritual world and the ethical standards societies apply to their members. The mentally ill, in their disorganized, agitated, or withdrawn states, are often both frightening and incomprehensible. It is understandable how such behavior could be attributed to spiritual possession. For all cultures, it has been a long journey to look for natural rather than supernatural explanations for illness. Witchcraft, deities, and the Devil have all been blamed for causing mental illness. Unfortunately, these views still exist throughout the world. The problem is not the belief in an evil or supernatural causation per se; rather, it is how that view of causation influences the care of the mentally ill. If an illness is thought to be caused by an evil spirit, does the society respond by persecuting, ostracizing, or even killing the affected individual? Or does the society respond by providing the best care and treatment its technology will allow? Can the society develop a naturalistic (i.e., clinical or scientific) approach that permits better understanding and treatment?

Enlightened views on the mentally ill were present in the early Christian hospitals, Buddhist missionaries, Confucian scholars, medieval Jewish physicians, and the Islamic hospitals of the Middle Ages. However, many societies had a flowering of enlightened care only to later revert to unscientific and sometimes inhumane practices. This regression was epitomized in the medieval Christian Inquisition, when many mentally ill individuals were identified as witches and killed. The true inspiration of the major religions—the wisdom of Confucius, the compassion of Buddha, the sense of justice of the Prophets, the love of Jesus, and the fair and skillful administration of Mohammed—guides our medical ethics. Our physician predecessors Hippocrates, Casaka, Chang Chung-Ching, Maimonides, Avicenna, and Weyer can guide our clinical work. Our challenge is to be worthy of our moral, intellectual, and clinical inheritance.

References

Al-Issa I: Psychiatry in Algeria. Psychiatric Bulletin 13:240–245, 1989

Al-Mutlaq H: Aspects of non-spiritual rewards of Islamic fundamentalism. Mind and Human Interaction 7:91–96, 1996

Al-Radi OM, Al-Mahdy MA: Group therapy: an Islamic approach. Transcultural Psychiatric Research Review 26:273–276, 1989

Al-Sabair A: Psychiatry in Saudi Arabia: cultural perspectives. Transcultural Psychiatric Research Review 26:245–262, 1989

Alexander FG, Selesnick ST: The History of Psychiatry: An Evaluation of Psychiatric Thought and Practice From Prehistoric Times to the Present. New York, Harper & Row, 1966

Allan N: Hospice to hospital in the Near East: an instance of continuity and change in late antiquity. Bull Hist Med 64:446–462, 1990

Armstrong K: A History of God: The 4000-Year Quest of Judaism, Christianity and Islam. New York, Alfred A Knopf, 1993

Atwood JD, Maltin L: Putting Eastern philosophies into Western psychotherapies. Am J Psychother 45:368–382, 1991

Baasher T: The Arab countries, in World History of Psychiatry. Edited by Howells JG. New York, Brunner/Mazel, 1975, pp 547–578

Ball RA, Clare AW: Symptoms and social adjustment in Jewish depressives. Br J Psychiatry 156:379–383, 1990

Bibal AM, Angelo-Khattan M: Correlates of alcohol-related casualties in Kuwait. Acta Psychiatr Scand 71:1–4, 1988

Bogart G: The use of meditation in psychotherapy: a review of the literature. Am J Psychother 45:383–412, 1991

Bromberg W: From Shaman to Psychotherapist: A History of the Treatment of Mental Illness. Chicago, IL, Henry Regnery, 1975

Chaudhry MR: The role of the mosque in mental health in psychiatry: a world perspective. Excerpta Medica Amsterdam 4:244–248, 1990

Dradkey TK: Parasuicide during Ramadan in Jordon. Acta Psychiatr Scand 86:253–254, 1992

Desjarlais R, Eisenberg L, Good B, et al: World Mental Health: Problems and Priorities in Low-Income Countries. New York, Oxford University Press, 1995

Dols MW (tr): Ibn Redwân's Treatise "On the Prevention of Bodily Ills in Egypt." Berkeley, CA, University of California Press, 1984

Dols MW: The origins of the Islamic hospital: myth and reality. Bull Hist Med 61:367–390, 1987a

Dols MW: Insanity and its treatment in Islamic society. Med Hist 31:1–14, 1987b

Epler DC: The concept of disease in an ancient Chinese medical text: the discourse on cold-camage disorders (Shang-han Lun). J Hist Med Allied Sci 43:8–35, 1988

Epstein M: Thoughts Without a Thinker: Psychotherapy From a Buddhist Perspective. New York, Basic Books, 1995

Favazza AR: Modern Christian healing of mental illness. Am J Psychiatry 139:728–735, 1982

Feldman DM: Health and Medicine in the Jewish Tradition. New York, Crossroad, 1986

Ferngren GB: Early Christianity as a religion of healing. Bull Hist Med 66:1–15, 1992

Frankl VE: Man's Search for Meaning: An Introduction to Logotherapy. New York, Washington Square Press, 1963

Freud S: Moses and monotheism (1939), in The Standard Edition of the Complete Psychological Works of Sigmund Freud, Vol 23. Translated and edited by Strachey J. London, Hogarth, 1964, pp 1–137

Funk RW, Hoover RW, and The Jesus Seminar: The Five Gospels: The Search for the Authentic Words of Jesus. New York, Macmillan, 1993

Graziani JS: Arabic Medicine in the Eleventh Century as Represented in the Works of Ibn Jazlah. Karachi, Pakistan, Handard Academy, 1980

Hajal F: Galen's ethical psychotherapy: its influence on a medieval Near East physician. J Hist Med Allied Sci 38:320–333, 1983

Hsu H-Y, Peacher WG: Shang Han Lun (The Great Classic of Chinese Medicine). Long Beach, CA, Oriental Healing Arts Institute, 1981

Ishimaru-Tseng TV: Morita therapy: good match for managed care? Psychiatric Times, September 1996, p 22

Kinzie JD, Goetz RR: A century of controversy surrounding posttraumatic stress-spectrum syndromes: the impact on DSM-III and DSM-IV. J Trauma Stress 9: 159–179, 1996

Knoll J, Bachrach B: Sin and mental illness in the Middle Ages. Psychol Med 14:507–514, 1984

Knoll J, Bachrach B: Sin and the etiology of disease in pre-Crusade Europe. J Hist Med Allied Sci 41:395–414, 1986

Leiser G: Medical education in Islamic lands from the seventh to the fourteenth century. J Hist Med Allied Sci 38:48–73, 1983

MacDonald M: Mystical Bedlam. Cambridge, UK, Cambridge University Press, 1981

Miles J: God: A Biography. New York, Alfred A Knopf, 1995

Miller L: Israel and the Jews, in World History of Religion. Edited by Howells JG. New York, Brunner/Mazel, 1975, pp 528–546

Mollica RF, Streets FJ, Boscarino J, et al: A community study of formal pastoral counseling activities of the clergy. Am J Psychiatry 143:323–328, 1986

Nozick R: The Examined Life: Philosophical Meditations. New York, Simon & Schuster, 1989

Pagels E: The Origins of Satan. New York, Random House, 1995

Rao AV: India, in World History of Psychiatry. Edited by Howells JG. New York, Brunner/Mazel, 1975, pp 624–649

Roohanna R: A pilot study of alcohol drinkers in Ahwaz, Iran. International Journal of the Addictions 21:399–410, 1986

Rosner F: Studies in Torah Judaism: Modern Medicine and Jewish Law. New York, Yishiva University, Department of Special Publications, 1972

Rosner F: Moses, Maimonides and preventive medicine. J Hist Med Allied Sci 51:313–324, 1996

Sauna VD: Mental illness and other forms of psychiatric deviance among contemporary Jewry. Transcultural Psychiatric Research Review 29:197–233, 1992

Shamasundar C: Therapeutic wisdom in Indian mythology. Am J Psychother 47:443–449, 1993

Simons RC, Ervin FR, Prince RH: The psychobiology of trance, parts I and II. Transcultural Psychiatric Research Review 25:249–284, 1988

Smith H: The World's Religions: Our Great Wisdom Traditions. San Francisco, CA, Harper, 1991

Thich Nhat Hanh: Old Path, White Clouds: Walking in the Footsteps of the Buddha. Berkeley, CA, Parallax Press, 1991

Tseng WS: The development of psychiatric concepts in traditional Chinese medicine. Arch Gen Psychiatry 29:569–575, 1973a

Tseng WS: The concept of personality in Confucian thought. Psychiatry 36:191–202, 1973b

Unschuld PU: Medical Ethics in Imperial China—A Study in Historical Anthropology. Berkeley, CA, University of California Press, 1979

Unschuld PU: Medicine in China: A History of Ideas. Berkeley, CA, University of California Press, 1985

Vahia NS, Vinekar SL, Doongaji DR: Some ancient Indian concepts in the treatment of psychiatric disorders. Br J Psychiatry 112:1089–1096, 1966

Veith I (tr): Huang Di Nei Ching Su Wen (The Yellow Emperor's Classic of Internal Medicine). Berkeley, CA, University of California Press, 1949

Veith I: The Far East: reflections on the psychological foundations, in World History of Psychiatry. Edited by Howells JG. New York, Brunner/Mazel, 1975, pp 662–703

Walsh R: Two Asian psychologies and their implications for Western psychotherapists. Am J Psychother 42:543–560, 1988

Wang SY, Hsu HY (tr): Chang Chung-Ching—Chin Kuli Yao Lulh: Prescriptions From the Golden Chamber. Long Beach, CA, Oriental Healing Arts Institute, 1983

Young A: The return of "The Return of the Repressed" (review essay). Transcultural Psychiatric Research Review 29:235–243, 1992

Zilboorg G: The Medical Man and the Witch During the Renaissance. Baltimore, MD, Johns Hopkins University Press, 1935

Zilboorg G: A History of Medical Psychology. New York, WW Norton, 1941

✿ CHAPTER 2 ✿

Psychiatry and Religion in Cross-Cultural Context

Charles C. Hughes, Ph.D.,[†] *and*
Ronald M. Wintrob, M.D.

Stripped to semantic essentials, the terms *religion* and *psychiatry* refer to antithetic yet complementary "realities" that illustrate the epistemological richness of the human experience. While both are products of the symbolizing power of the evolved neocortex, psychiatry asserts that the only valid source of knowledge is the observable world, and the discipline's conceptualizations and therapeutic activities are based on a scientific approach to understanding. Like science, religious thought is also grounded in that evolutionary attribute—the ability to "make" a world (Goodman 1978)—but it is programmed by essentially different premises. In the case of religion, that "world" is constructed not of what presumably *is*, but of what *could* or *might be—a subjunctive world*, a world of myth and imagination, of " . . . if only it *were* the case that . . . ." Northrop's characterization of the contrasting epistemological groundings of science and religion is helpful in understanding their differences in "worldview." *Existential* beliefs are assertions about the nature of the empirical world based on investigation of that world—*about what is*—whereas *normative* beliefs are assertions about *what should be, ought to be*, and *is wished to be* (Northrop 1949, pp. 256–257). The phenomenology of human life attests to the profound importance of each "reality" in serving fundamental needs in both personal and social life.

[†]Deceased.

Given the renewed interest of the medical profession in relations between religion (or "spirituality"), medicine, and psychiatry, an exploration of the interplay between religion and psychiatry has become a timely theoretical—as well as pragmatic—issue. After decades in which scientific skepticism and Freudian disapproval have kept religion at a polite distance from medicine, a door between the two fields has opened (Condon 1995). As noted in Chapter 9 of this volume, guidelines for the teaching of the importance of religion and spirituality in clinical practice have been incorporated in new accreditation guidelines for psychiatry residency training programs.

In June 1996, *Time* magazine carried a lengthy article that discussed several empirically grounded studies of the purported power of prayer and religion in promoting healing. Also in 1996, the journal *Science* included a review article concerning a number of experiments designed to study the healing potential of prayer (Thomson 1996). Many studies of this subject can be faulted for the limited range of empirical data used to examine the presumed relationship. Typically, the religious variable in the proposed relationship is phrased solely in terms of culturally Eurocentric references to "God," thus ignoring many other cultural conceptions of which deity or deities should be considered, as well as the ubiquitous spiritualized forces of nature found in many of the world's religions. Would the same purported effects obtain if prayer were directed at one of the major figures in the pantheon of Hindu deities? Or, as in China or many African societies, to one's ancestors? Thus, if the research issue is the relationship between the cultural construct "religion" and healing, it is imperative that a cross-cultural perspective be applied.

Another question that goes to the heart of the topic of this chapter is whether the relationship between "religion" and "healing" is *causal* or simply *correlational?* Are "cures" or the alleviation of suffering attributable to a transempirical "power" directing secular human affairs, or are they instead due to patients' *beliefs* that through prayer a desired outcome will be achieved? Herbert Benson, author of *Timeless Healing: The Power and Biology of Belief* (1996), has long been concerned with the healing powers of the mind. Rousch (1997), in a recent article reviewing Benson's work, commented that "the very act of believing—no matter what our religion or philosophy—can help keep us well." In another recent assessment of this subject, Baker (1997) stated:

> What I'm saying . . . [is that] it is not that faith heals, but that belief heals, and the belief may or may not be religious. (p. 20)

The purpose of this chapter is to explore the intellectual and pragmatic dialectics between religion—as conceptualized and illustrated in a highly selective sampling of its great institutional variety in human cultures—and psychiatry and related forms of psychosocial and psychobiological healing (e.g., Csordas and Kleinman 1996; Dow 1986). That is no simple task. As Ventis (1995) has noted:

> In approaching the study of the relationship between religion and mental health, we would do well to remember the fable of the three blind men and the elephant. In this story, each man, not being able to see the animal, touched a different part (e.g., the tail, the side, the trunk) and drew completely different, overly simple, and only partially valid conclusions about the nature of the beast. Meanwhile, each assumed that he had a completely adequate grasp of the subject. These three blind men were actually fairly fortunate because they had only one complex subject to try to understand. In our consideration of religion and mental health, we are confronted with two. (p. 33)

Notwithstanding differences in underlying ethos, psychiatry and religion share several structural and terminological features. For one thing, although different in content, their conceptualizations have a common source—*human behavior*—and that behavioral base is the locus of the problems and issues with which they both deal: the perplexities, frustrations, disorders, mysteries, anxieties, and fears of daily life. Yet even as it functions as a *cause* of problems, each domain also provides its own distinctive modes of explanation, relief, and resolution of life's problems. Thus, for example, in psychiatry there is a *diagnosis*—an intellectual formulation of a given problem—and recommended treatments to effect its resolution (e.g., punitive childhood socialization experience, with psychotherapy as a possible mode of resolution). In religion, breaking a taboo might be advanced as the cause of an affliction, and confession, the "treatment" advised for its resolution.

Another feature psychiatry and religion have in common is the use of three descriptive terms that serve very different functions in each institutional area: "belief," "spirituality," and "possession"—terms that can lead the unwary to assume similar *meanings* in both contexts. Although the terms used are different in each domain, a common psychological process is significantly involved in the workings of both religion and psychiatry: the familiar "placebo effect."

Belief

Behavior is the naturalistic source of a concept—*belief*—that is crucial to both religion and psychiatry but takes on different operational characteristics and claims to validity in each:

> Beliefs are propositions about the relations among things to which those who
> believe have made some kind of commitment. Commitment may be for prag-
> matic or emotional reasons. A proposition's credibility may appear obvious
> from experience, or a proposition may seem to be the most prudent assumption
> on which to act. In either case, the commitment has a pragmatic basis. Emo-
> tional commitment to a proposition occurs when a person wants or feels a need
> for it to be true because of what its truth implies about things that matter.
> (Goodenough 1990, p. 597)

But that abstract conceptual vessel *belief* can be filled with different empirical contents. In religion, beliefs refer to presumed entities, events, and
processes in a *supernatural world*. In psychiatry, belief statements are conceptualized in a positivistic, empirical, "scientific" frame of reference.

Spirituality

Another term—though not necessarily the same concept—used by both religion and psychiatry is *spirituality*—often referred to but never defined opera-
tionally in terms that would satisfy an empiricist, which is a difficulty
acknowledged by some authors; for example:

> . . . a vernacular in which to address the concept of spiritual well-being is not
> without its problems either, because at best human spirituality is ineffable. In
> other words, we don't possess the vocabulary to give this concept an adequate
> definition or description. (Seaward 1995, p. 166)

A term often used interchangeably with spirituality is *faith*. Spirituality
may be taken as a concept that quintessentially refers to a "religious" domain.
Yet examples of published definitions implicitly suggest a relationship between the behavioral *sciences* and religion:

> As a working definition, we propose that *spirituality* entails the acknowledge-
> ment of a transcendent being, power, or reality greater than ourselves . . . . Fur-
> thermore, spirituality involves an attempt to align and conform one's own life
> (both covert and overt behavior) toward this higher power. (Miller and Martin
> 1988, p. 14)

> By "spirituality," I point toward the transcendence of human morality I
> refer specifically to the notion of the supernatural . . . . (Pattison 1988, p. 184)

> For many people, the term *spirituality* has otherworldly connotations and im-
> plies some form of religious discipline. The term is used here in a broad sense,

however, to refer to the ultimate values and meanings in terms of which we live, whether they be otherworldly or very worldly ones, and whether or not we consciously try to increase our commitment to those values and meanings. The term does have religious connotations, in that one's ultimate values and meanings reflect some presupposition as to what is *holy*, that is, of ultimate importance. (Griffin 1988, p. 1)

It is important to mark the use of several terms and phrases—"acknowledgement of a transcendent being"; "an attempt to align and conform one's own life (both covert and overt behavior) toward this higher power"; "notion of the supernatural"; "the ultimate values and meanings in terms of which we live"—again, all within the semantic realm of *belief* as scientifically conceptualized.

The term *spirituality* is Janus-like, bridging the two domains of religion and science; indeed, when a serious attempt at definition is made, the language employed usually consists of empirically assessable operational indicators. For example:

> The construct of the human spirit can be described best as integration of three facets: an insightful relationship with oneself and others, a strong personal value system, and a meaningful purpose to one's life. (Seaward 1991, p. 167)

In addition to being a signal marker of "religion," spirituality is also often taken as an important "variable" in an empirically based analysis of the human predicament (Lukoff et al. 1992, 1995). Religious beliefs and practices may provide solace and solutions to numerous problems of living, but adherence to religious beliefs can also *create* conflict, guilt, and fear (Patel 1995). For example, difficulties associated with religious faith or spiritual values are included in the DSM-IV category "religious or spiritual problem" (V62.89 [American Psychiatric Association 1994, p. 685]). The following case exemplifies such a problem:

> Ms. L, a woman of Irish-Catholic background in her mid-30s, was recently treated by one of the authors (RW). The youngest of three siblings, the woman had a distant relationship with her older brother, an attorney, who she felt had been responsible for her involuntary hospitalization during a period of depression following the breakup of her marriage several years earlier. The relationship with her much older sister had been very close—more like that with a surrogate mother—until her sister left home, when Ms. L was 8 years old, to become a nun. In recent years, it had been expected by the patient's siblings (and by Ms. L herself) that she would live with her widowed and ill mother,

who, Ms. L felt, had never given her the recognition, approval, and affection that her two older (and, in her mother's eyes, more successful) siblings had been given.

Ms. L. felt increasingly stifled and overburdened by the demands of looking after her mother, both because of her mother's declining health and because of her intensely ambivalent feelings toward her mother. She became increasingly withdrawn, angry, irritable, and depressed. As these symptoms intensified, so did feelings of self-blame and guilt about her wish to escape the responsibilities of living with and caring for her mother. She became very preoccupied with feelings of personal failure/culpability for the breakup of her marriage and for having had an abortion 2 years prior to her marriage. She became convinced that she deserved divine punishment and thought that suicide would be her only means of relief. Soon after that, she reported that the walls of her bedroom seemed to glow and that the saints and possibly also "the divine spirit" were influencing her thoughts and guiding her behavior. She became overtalkative and agitated and, after a highly inappropriate verbal outburst during a church service, was referred for urgent psychiatric assessment.

As this case illustrates, stressful life events can transform some patients' normative religious beliefs into excessive religious preoccupations, often involving self-blame and guilt over real or imagined religious transgressions. Further stress can lead to psychotic distortions involving religious themes. Very depressed patients may feel that by their (self-assessed) acts of nastiness to others (e.g., behaving irresponsibly toward family, co-workers, or members of social groups to which they belong) they have caused grievous harm and should be punished by God for their transgressions or that they should kill themselves, because their moral transgressions are too serious to be forgotten by those they have wronged or by God.

Psychopathological distortion of normative religious beliefs can also be seen in schizophrenic patients, some of whom believe, during the prodromal/early stages of their illness, that special powers have been given to them by divine sources and that they can use these powers to influence other people's actions or the outcome of events affecting their families, fellow workers, or communities. In the more florid stages of the illness, patients may believe that they hear God talking to them and guiding their actions.

"Possession"

Although the term *possession* is in the lexicons of both psychiatry and religion, it has quite different ideational and ontological implications in each. In religion, a person may be possessed by some otherworldly force (e.g., the spirit of an ancestor or deity, a malevolent spirit, or the Holy Ghost); in psychiatry, possession is by an alternative personality, as in the dissociative fragmentation of the personality (Kenney 1981). As a psychological process and ritual enactment, possession is a phenomenon that can be observed and studied worldwide, reflecting both personal and social values (Crapanzano and Garrison 1977; Oesterreich 1966).

The Placebo Effect

Regardless of its specific content, the operative power of belief provides another example of a common feature found in both religion and psychiatry—the *placebo effect*. This term refers to the often-dramatic consequences for behavior change and restructuring of belief energized by involvement in a ritually defined social context in which the participants share a common system of ideas (Frank and Frank 1993). Speaking of non-Western healing systems, Moerman (1983) noted the significance of the placebo effect in commenting that " . . . neither native therapists nor their patients saw pharmaceuticals as any more important in therapy than the song, dance, and din that accompanied treatment" (p. 156). He expressed the issue well in the succinct phrase "meaning mends" (Moerman 1983, p. 164).

Prince (1976) referred to the "self-healing mechanisms" involved in ritual healing as "endogenous" processes that occur in the context of the symbol-laden theater of a "religious" event:

> . . . under conditions of stress, individuals have resorted to a repertoire of automatic self-healing mechanisms. The most important of these are so-called altered states of consciousness—dreams, dissociated states, a variety of religious experiences, and . . . the psychotic reactions . . . . [Many] of the healing techniques used around the world are simply manipulations and elaborations of these endogenous healing mechanisms. (p. 116)

Consistent with Prince and with the analysis offered by Ness and Wintrob (1981) about the numerous therapeutic aspects of traditional healing patterns, Harding (1975) further noted that

> in many cultures the healer is at one and the same time a religious leader in touch with the ancestors and the spirit world and a doctor who concerns himself with the sick and disabled. (p. 437)

Psychosocial and Religious "Healing": Examples

Shamanism

Perhaps the first form of "religion" in human history was the ancient and still widespread practice of *shamanism,* common to many cultures, in which the healer undergoes a dissociative, ecstatic experience in the course of divination and treatment of the supplicant's disorder. The shaman's duties are several: alleviation of symptoms, "cure" of illness, and resolution of both individual and community quandaries (e.g., lack of rainfall that threatens drought and crop failure, unpredictable availability of an animal prey normally found, anxieties occasioned by an outbreak of witchcraft). Although the term *shamanism* has become popularized in modern society to the extent that it is often taken as any form of induced otherworldly experience (e.g., there are weekend urban workshops in "shamanizing"), the designation originally came from a Paleo-Siberian group, the Tungus (Lommel 1967; Shirokogoroff 1935; Walsh 1990), who used it to refer to a person (usually male) whose "soul" or spirit was believed able to leave the body and interact with the "other" world as the intermediary between the mundane problems of members of the community and the realm of the supernatural.

An example from the Siberian Eskimos can serve to illustrate the principal features of this widespread and ancient socioreligious complex. The aspiring shaman typically underwent a "vision-seeking" experience (i.e., a Vision Quest) in which he (or she) left the village settlement and endured a period of self-imposed denial of food and water, as well as exposure to the severe weather conditions of the frozen, windswept tundra. Having demonstrated such self-sacrifice, the aspiring shaman would then be visited by spirits, with whom he negotiated to help in the discovery/diagnostic and healing rituals that would subsequently be undertaken. In this group (the St. Lawrence Island Eskimos of the north Bering Sea), it was believed there were two types of spiritual entities—one that was relatively benign and amenable to helping humans, and another that was clearly malevolent and caused misfortune, illness, accidents, and death. The shaman's task was to enter that mysterious world of dangerous spirits and powerful supernatural forces, divine the cause of the "presenting problem," and—with the assistance of his spiritual helpers—overcome the malevolent spirit(s).

Clearly, in this behavioral pattern of shamanistic practice, no seam divided "religion" and "healing." The underlying rationale for the etiology of the problem as well as for the therapeutic process undertaken by the shaman was dictated by the belief system shared by the shaman and members of the community. The shaman's invocation of powerful spiritual agents, malevolent as well as benevolent, derived from religion but—in an empirical framework— functioned as a healing mechanism. Of special importance, not only the patient but also the patient's family participated in the healing ceremony, a highly ritualized sequence incorporating theatrical elements such as special costuming and instrumentation (e.g., drumming and dancing), ventriloquism and use of archaic language, dramatic explanations of the "cause" (typically the flight or theft of the patient's "soul"), and special behavioral prescriptions and proscriptions for the patient and the patient's family.

In order to create an atmosphere of confidence and readiness to believe, one renowned shaman was especially known for his ability to be resurrected from an apparent death-producing experience. Two strong men would pull the ends of a walrus-hide tether wrapped around his neck until there was the sound of a loud crack—as of the neck breaking—and, in the darkened room, of a body falling to the floor, lifeless. But shortly the shaman arose to resume the healing scenario. An important part of the therapeutic procedure was his using a bird's wing to brush the patient's body (thereby "brushing" away the malevolent spirits). Another technique was his touching or sucking on the patient's body and, after having done so, spitting out a bloody "worm" or other object that represented the sickness-causing agent (Hughes 1955). (In this connection, one notes the importance of touch and of brushing the patient's body with the raven's wing [Montagu 1971]).

Shamanistic practices are not limited to indigenous peoples living in isolated locations or in premodern times. Tobin and Friedman (1983) reported on the illness and healing of a Hmong refugee from Laos who was trying to cope with the profound stress of relocation to a strange country and way of life in the United States, following his family's escape from the turmoil of war-torn Laos. Five months after Vang, a 22-year-old Hmong man, arrived with his family in the United States and settled in Chicago, he began to experience progressively severe insomnia and frequent nightmares. On waking from his nightmares, Vang felt acute anxiety, fear of impending doom, shortness of breath, and chest pain. Vang's family consulted with elders of the Hmong community in Chicago, who recommended treatment by a traditional Hmong shaman. The shaman, Mrs. Thor,

. . . began by asking Vang to tell her what was wrong. She listened to his story, asked a few questions, and then told him she thought she could help. She gathered Vang's family around the dining room table, upon which she placed some candles alongside many plates of food that Vang's wife had prepared. Mrs. Thor lit the candles and then began a chant that Vang and his wife knew was an attempt to communicate with spirits. Ten minutes or so after Mrs. Thor had begun chanting, she was so intensely involved in her work that Vang and his family felt free to talk to each other and to walk about the room without fear of distracting her. Approximately 1 hour after she had begun, Mrs. Thor completed her chanting, announcing that she knew what was wrong. She said that she had learned from her spirit that the figures in Vang's dreams who lay on his chest and who made it so difficult for him to breathe were the souls of the apartment's [Vang's apartment] previous tenants, who had apparently moved out so abruptly that they had left their souls behind. Mrs. Thor constructed a cloak out of newspaper for Vang to wear. She then cut the cloak in two, and burned the pieces, sending the spirits on their way with the smoke. She also had Vang crawl through a hoop, and then between two knives, telling him that these maneuvers would make it very hard for spirits to follow. Following these brief ceremonies, the food prepared by Vang's wife was enjoyed by all. The leftover meats were given in payment to Mrs. Thor, and she left, assuring Vang that his troubles with spirits were over. (Tobin and Friedman 1983, p. 441)

Tobin and Friedman's commentary on this case history succinctly expresses how cultural beliefs serve as the instrument of a transcultural psychotherapeutic process:

Mrs. Thor interpreted Vang's nightmares and night breathing difficulties as, literally, spiritual problems. And since Vang, like Mrs. Thor, and indeed like virtually all Hmong, believes in spirits, her interpretations and ministrations on his behalf were intelligible, desired, and ultimately successful. (Tobin and Friedman 1983, p. 441)

Tobin and Friedman also noted that cases similar to Vang's in symptomatology and affecting previously healthy young adults have had fatal outcomes, and that postmortem examination could not identify the cause of death. These cases have come to be called "Hmong sudden-death syndrome" (Tobin and Friedman 1983, p. 440).

Priestly Healing

Whereas shamanistic practices and beliefs typically emphasize the dissociative, highly individualized performances of the healer, in many other societies the predominant form of "religious" healer is the priest, who enacts rites that are highly scripted (Turner 1968).

Navajo. The healing and religious beliefs and practices of the Navajo Indians provide an example of priestly healing and illness causation. Navajo religion comprises a complex catalog of situations and actions a person must avoid, lest illness be the outcome. There is an extensive body of beliefs dictating avoidance of many kinds of dangerous objects or situations *(báhádzid—* "dangerous to do")*;* for example, coming into contact with a tree or anything that had been struck by lightning could cause major symptoms of distress, as will seeing a coyote or entering a *hogan* (traditional dwelling) where someone has died (Kluckhohn and Leighton 1948; Leighton and Leighton 1941, 1945; Reichard 1945). Infractions of such specific proscriptions are post hoc explanations for illness and "dys-ease" affecting both the transgressor and his or her family. Furthermore, they are manifestations of a more pervasive concept, that of being "out of harmony" with the universe; indeed, the idea of " . . . *hózhó,* [is] the most important concept in traditional Navajo culture, which combines the concepts of beauty, goodness, order, harmony, and everything that is positive or ideal" (Carrese and Rhodes 1995, p. 826).

The purpose of the complex healing ceremonies is to restore a person's sense of total well-being and rectitude—in short, the feeling that one is "in harmony" once again with the universe. The healing ceremonies—one of which, the major ceremony "Blessing Way," lasts 9 days—are conducted by priest-healers called "Singers"; they include chanting of lengthy mythic texts and incorporate other ceremonial features, with members of the patient's family and clan in attendance. Navajo ceremonialism is highly prescriptive, with deviation from the memorized "texts" resulting in failure to achieve the goal of alleviating the problem, thereby placing the individual, family, and clan at further risk of misfortune and illness.

Yoruba. Prince (1964) has noted the close relationship between religion and healing among the Yoruba people of Nigeria, where the chief healer is also of the priestly tradition. Speaking of one aspect of the highly complex Yoruba religion, he described the diffuse way in which religious concepts constitute both etiology and therapy:

> . . . [When] a man falls ill, he will first try a home remedy or one purchased from an itinerant medicine peddler. If he does not recover, he may consult a *babalawo* (traditional priest-healer) who, after divination, will advise that he make a sacrifice to the witches, his double, his ancestors or one of the *Orisas* [deities]; take certain medicines or use certain magical devices for protection against sorcerers, witches, or bad spirits; change his place of abode (because of the witches in the compound) or, more rarely, change his occupation (because

he is not fulfilling his heavenly contract); change his character—be less aggressive, proud, impatient, and so forth; take a medicine for disease of the body; become an initiate into one of the *Orisa* cults (generally one's lineage *Orisa* or one that was formerly in one's lineage, although this association may have been forgotten by living members and may be discovered only by divination). (Prince 1964, pp. 104–105).

Reference to the religious healing of the Yoruba people is especially relevant in this context, since many of the African slaves brought to the New World belonged to the Yoruba tribe and had been enculturated into the Yoruba belief system. The names and concepts of their spiritual entities (e.g., *orisa*, a general term for deity) have been incorporated into the candomblé practices and voodoo beliefs of Brazil, the Caribbean, and other Central and South American countries.

Spirit Possession and Malign Magic

Given the ubiquity of religious beliefs and practices that are built upon the notion of possession, trance, and "unusual mental states," and the obvious relevance of those practices for psychiatry (Bourguignon 1966, 1976; Kiev 1972), this topic will be examined in its ethnographic variations in several parts of the world.

Africa

From the Muslim Maghreb of North Africa to sub-Saharan animistic, Muslim, and Christian West African countries, the cultural diffusion of belief in possession by spirits has been very extensive. In the traditional beliefs of the Maghreb, the spirit world is pervasive in daily life and family interactions, and the risk of possession by a playful or malevolent spirit is an everyday source of caution and concern (Crapanzano 1973, 1975; Wintrob 1977). Since unreasonable jealousy of the accomplishments of others in the community is believed to be in itself a provocation of the spirit world, widespread belief in susceptibility to possession by punitive spirits can serve as a powerful inducement to and reinforcement of harmonious interpersonal relationships. But given the inevitability of envy and resentment in human interrelatedness, it is seen as inevitable that retribution can always occur—for example, in the form of possession by malevolent spirits. In the North African Maghreb, such spirits are called "djinns" or "jnun," and in West Africa, "djinni" or "genii" (Wintrob 1966).

Although the consequences of possession by malevolent djinns are thought to vary greatly, the predominant description encompasses a full range of neuropsychiatric phenomena, including faintness and fainting spells, obtunding or loss of consciousness, tremor, weakness, restlessness or agitation, outbursts of irritability or aggressiveness, assaultiveness or destruction of property, insomnia, distractibility and inability to concentrate, emotional lability, social withdrawal, and bizarre speech that reflects disorganized thought processes, delusions, and hallucinations (Crapanzano 1973; Wintrob 1966). If a community member is at the more severe end of the scale of disturbance of psychological functioning, all concerned members of the "victim's" family and community recognize the need for specialized treatment to relieve the obvious distress.

In such cases, help is sought from a spiritual healer who almost always has the status of a religious authority; the healer's ascribed power is thought to derive directly from his or her role as an intermediary between the spirit world and the world of humans. The authority, the social status, and the healing power of these special people are gradually acquired through the cumulative record of their perceived success in calming the troubled spirits of their supplicants; by their success in enticing, cajoling, or outwitting the troublesome spirits and inducing them to leave the victim completely; or by diminishing or neutralizing the disturbing influence of these spirits on the victim (Prince 1964; Wintrob 1966).

By their very nature, healing ceremonies of this kind are religious and communal, involving public demonstration of the healer's powers. The locus is either a healing shrine or the victim's home, with the victim being accompanied and attended by extended family and community supporters. The healing ceremonies are dramatic in their intensity and protracted in their duration.

Following recovery of the victim, ritualistic ceremonies are instituted over many months to prevent return of the offending spirits and ensure the victim's recovery of prior familial, social, and occupational roles and status relationships. Important to the achievement of these aspects of recovery and of social acceptance is the victim's—and family's—participation in a healing group composed of experienced and high-status healers, their assistants, and people who, like the victim, are in the process of recovery or have recently recovered from possession by troublesome spirits. The mutual support of the members of these "healing cults" and the promise such groups hold for victims to accrue status in the cult and in the community by progressing from victim to recoverer, assistant healer, and finally healer are powerful reinforcers of recovery and social acceptance (Prince 1976; Wintrob 1973).

Caribbean and South American Cultures

The spread of traditions of beliefs in spirit possession and malign magic from Africa to the Caribbean and the Americas has been repeatedly documented (e.g., Sereno 1948). One example is the Orisa cult of the Yoruba people of Nigeria; it is found in places such as Trinidad, and the observances are strikingly similar to those in Nigeria (Mischel and Mischel 1958)

Perhaps the best known and most dramatic example of spirit possession rituals in the New World is that of "voodoo" (a term reportedly derived from *vodun*, a West African deity) in Haiti and elsewhere in the Caribbean (Kiev 1961; Mischel and Mischel 1958) and even in the contemporary United States (Maduro 1975). In this widely encountered tradition, it is believed that the bodies and minds of supplicants at a voodoo ritual can be temporarily possessed—or "ridden by the gods" or spirits—in much the same way as a rider controls the horse. Those who join in the voodoo rituals do so in the hope that being "ridden by the gods" will relieve them of misfortune, illness, or grief that has overtaken them and/or their family (Kiev 1966).

Voodoo ceremonies are conducted by spirit priest-healers known as *houngans*, most of whom have spent years learning the cosmology of voodoo beliefs and rituals essential to fulfilling their ceremonial as well as their healing roles. The knowledge and skills are generally passed down through generations of priest-healer families, such that the authority and reputation of many *houngans* is legendary. Since voodoo rituals often last for several days, and preparation for them may require several more days, they are viewed as community events of great importance.

Fundamental to voodoo belief are the characteristics of the possessing spirits or gods *(loas)*, who are thought to select for possession only those individuals most in need of their intervention and most compatible with them. The characteristics of the *loas* are quite specific: one is believed to be mischievous, playful, willful, and irresponsible; another is subject to sudden changes of mood, with intense outbursts of anger and aggression alternating with sympathy and soothing; another is very erotic and prone to sexual excess; and still another is described as avenging wrongs.

An essential element of voodoo ritual is the evocation of the *loas* through trance. Voodoo priests and their assistants are expected to prove their communion with the gods by entering into trance, during which they frequently speak in tongues and show some of the defining behavioral and temperamental characteristics of the spirits. Having achieved such a state of oneness with the spirit world, the voodoo priests and their assistants then help some of those among the supplicants to enter trance states, to commune with the spirits, and to be "mounted" by the particular spirit needed by that suppli-cant. The entire process is accompanied by intense dancing, drumming, music, prayer, burning of incense, invocation of the spirits, and the dramatic evidence of priest-healers, their assistants, and supplicants entering into trance and behav-ing in the ways defined by their possessing spirits. After coming out of trance, the supplicant subsides into exhaustion and is supported and cared for by the *houngan*'s assistants as well as by the supplicant's family and friends. To be cho-sen by the gods—to be ridden by their spirits—is regarded as a mark of distinc-tion in the community. It is equally viewed as a means of transferring supplicants' problems, illnesses, and misfortunes onto the gods—and by so do-ing, relieving supplicants of the intensity of their worries.

United States

Healing rituals related to spirit possession and malign magic can be found throughout the United States, reflecting the great diversity of ethnic back-grounds and religious traditions of the country. For illustrative purposes, two examples are described here: Fundamentalist Christian "faith healing" and "rootwork."

Faith healing.   In Fundamentalist Christian religious practices, such as those described by LaBarre (1962; Appalachian Pentecostal ceremonies), Csordas (1983; [southeastern United States), Pattison and Wintrob (1981; common elements of faith healing), and Ness and Wintrob (1980; northeast-ern United States and Newfoundland [Canada]), both minister and congrega-tion may fervently attest their purity of spirit by giving accounts of their previous experiences of "possession by the Holy Spirit." In particularly dra-matic displays of faith, as seen, for example, in Appalachia, the minister and some congregants will provide further demonstration of their profound trust in the goodness and protectiveness of the Holy Spirit—and, by inference, its protective infusion of themselves—by grasping and holding in front of them one or more large, poisonous snakes while they recount their past and present faith and good works in the service of the Lord, secure in the conviction that their faith will prevent them from being bitten.

Pentecostal healing ceremonies share many features with the African, Ca-ribbean, and South American religious healing traditions described in this chapter. These common elements include the following:

- Dramatic attestations and demonstrations of the past and recent powers of the minister/healer to achieve spiritual healing personally and on behalf of members of the congregation

- Ability of the minister/healer to serve as the medium for "the Divine Spirit" by going into trance during healing ceremonies and speaking in tongues
- Ability of the minister/healer to encourage and elicit attestations of profound faith in congregants, such that some congregants will themselves enter into a trance state and become possessed by "the Holy Spirit"
- Attestations by congregants to the effectiveness of "faith healing," not only by accounts of relief of symptoms of anxiety, depression, and despair; disordered and/or abusive behavior; or excessive drinking or family conflict, but also by accounts of their and their family members' recovery from serious physical disorders without the need of medical intervention.

Rootwork. Rootwork comprises a set of beliefs and practices closely linked to Caribbean voodoo. Although it is encountered principally in the southeastern United States, migration trends during the past several generations have had the effect of carrying rootwork traditions north and west through much of the eastern half of the country (Snow 1974; Tinling 1967; Wintrob 1973).

The underlying premises of rootwork center on the belief that any individual who is jealous and resentful of the accomplishments of another may, through the invocation of malign magic, cause misfortune, illness, or even death to befall the envied person. Among those who share such beliefs, relief from the "placing of a spell"—of *"being rooted"*—requires the help and active intervention of a *rootworker*—an individual believed to possess magical powers to both invoke and remove evil spells. Rootworkers are well known in their communities and are seen as combining the characteristics of religious healers and alternative medical healers (i.e., non-M.D.'s).

The social conflict most likely to engender accusations of rootwork involves a love triangle in which the rejected lover may claim that the successful lover has "placed a spell" on him or her in order to break his or her romantic hold over the person they both desire.

Alternatively, the rejected lover may be suspected of having had a spell placed on the person he or she loved and lost, as punishment for the rejection. The consequences of being victimized by such malign magic are believed to be inevitable and to include both physical and psychological suffering. Prominent among the psychological consequences of "being rooted" are anxiety; agitation; social withdrawal; inability to concentrate; feelings of hopelessness and impending doom; a precipitous decline in sleep, appetite, self-esteem, and coping ability; and, often enough, psychotic disorganization.

Consultation with a rootworker is done privately, with only the supplicant and one or two relatives and friends meeting with the healer. The rootworker usually gathers information from the supplicant and accompanying individuals about the victim's recent life history and important interpersonal relationships, paying particular attention to stressors and rivalrous interactions. Having done this, and sometimes also communing with the spirit world to further discern the causes of the supplicant's distress, the rootworker generally prescribes a regimen of daily prayers, sacrifices, and proscriptions against performing a range of activities that could endanger the victim or exacerbate the situation. The rootworker him- or herself offers prayers and incantations to neutralize the effects of the spell or evil spirits to which the supplicant is believed to have fallen victim. It is understood that particularly powerful rootworkers are capable not only of neutralizing the effects of an evil spell but also of returning the spell to its perpetrator, with the result that the perpetrator may be overtaken by the same misfortunes that had been intended for the victim of the original spell.

Syncretism

It would be simplistic to consider that a "religion" is always a self-contained, historically and internally consistent set of beliefs and practices. Indeed, in human affairs, diffusion, "borrowing," and incorporation of formerly alien traits have been universal.

Fusion of animistic, Muslim, and Christian religions.   Liberia, in West Africa, offers good examples of such phenomena in the syncretism of animistic, Muslim, and Christian traditions of its diverse population. During the years that one of the authors (RW) was that country's only psychiatrist (many years before the tragic civil war that has engulfed the country since the late 1980s), nearly all patients who came or were brought to the attention of psychiatric services explained their illnesses as the direct result of witchcraft, spirit possession, or soul loss. The most common explanation was witchcraft—or, more specifically, victimization through malign magic inflicted by relatives, friends, or others in the community who were envious of the victim's (or his or her family's) achievements and status. It was the widely accepted belief that under such circumstances, jealous or evil-minded individuals could perpetrate an evil spell on the envied and/or resented person, usually through appeal to a prophet-healer who was believed to have the power to communicate with the spirit world. If the prophet-healer could be persuaded of the legitimacy of the supplicant's story, malevolent spirits or witches could be invoked. The result was believed to be that the victim of such witchcraft would soon lose his or her social advantages and become severely ill, in the same way as described for possession by malevolent djinns. In one such case,

> Rev. B, the 60-year-old minister of a Fundamentalist Christian church in the capital city, came for help because of the worsening of his distressing symptoms was. Married, a father, and a grandfather, Rev. B had been the pastor of his congregation for more than 20 years. He was, for all of these reasons, a man of high social status in the community in which he lived.
>
> During the year before he sought psychiatric help, Rev. B had been experiencing increasing urinary symptoms: dysuria, sometimes having blood-tinged urine, and increasing frequency of urination. His anxiety had greatly increased, and he had recently begun to have some urinary incontinence. He had not sought medical help because of embarrassment about his symptoms. As the symptoms became more acute, and especially as Rev. B became very fearful that his parishioners might notice his urinary incontinence, he began to ruminate about his condition. He began to think that something "unnatural" was afflicting him. Eventually, Rev. B became convinced that someone in his congregation had become so envious of him—of his reputation and status in the church and in the community—that he or she had "poisoned" him—that is, worked witchcraft on him. Ultimately, Rev. B felt certain that the perpetrator of his psychological torment and obvious physical illness had for years been throwing a "poison powder" in his path, in front of his house, and on the pathway to the minister's entrance to his church.
>
> Rev. B became very withdrawn, guarded in his interaction with his family and his parishioners, and subject to crying spells and unprovoked outbursts of anger. He felt unable to carry on with his ministry. Although he informed his wife that he thought he might be losing his mind, Rev. B told her nothing about his physical condition of dysuria and related symptoms. His wife knew about the mental health services in the capital and arranged an appointment for him. He was agitated and emotionally labile on assessment. He wept on several occasions, expressed shame and remorse, and told the following story:
>
>> Early on in his ministry with the current congregation, Rev. B had been attracted to one of the female parishioners. They had regular contact in connection with the conduct of his ministry, but for more than 10 years their contact had developed into an intimate relationship that both of them had been able to keep discreet. Rev. B felt that during the past year, his developing physical discomfort and symptoms of dysuria and recent incontinence were evidence of punishment by God for his deceitful and profoundly immoral behavior. He had become increasingly worried that he might be experiencing some sort of sexually transmitted illness, but this conviction made him feel so humiliated and ashamed of his sinful be-

havior that he told no one and avoided seeing a doctor. Ultimately, both his avoidance of help and his guilt about his behavior over the preceding 10 years overwhelmed him, and as he became more emotionally disturbed, Rev. B reinterpreted his symptoms in the conceptual framework he called "African science," or witchcraft inflicted on him by a jealous parishioner.

Following both physical and psychiatric treatment, the minister determined to end the relationship with his parishioner and to keep the whole affair secret from his family and church officials.

Candomblé.   Another example of syncretism is the candomblé ritual practices of Brazil, especially in the area of Bahia (Omwari 1984), where it is often said that there are no nonbelievers in "candomblé," only believers of greater or lesser intensity. Candomblé encompasses a set of beliefs in the power of the spirit world to relieve human suffering—a set of beliefs that incorporates an enormous and elaborate pantheon of gods and possessing spirits derived from African, Caribbean, and indigenous Brazilian tribal heritages, along with traditional European-derived religious movements. It is a form of syncretized informal religion that has a strong healing component.

Candomblé rituals are most often conducted in churches and community centers. They are viewed by their adherents as opportunities to make contact with the spirit world as a means of relieving anxiety; coping with and overcoming loss, grief, and personal misfortune; and atoning for wrongdoing, as well as a source of guidance for handling the stresses of family problems.

Adherents of candomblé are not limited to the poor and working-class population, nor to people whose main religious affiliation is Fundamentalist Christian. Rather, Candomblé is as universally held a belief and practice in Brazil as the annual month-long national preoccupation with the revelries of "Carnival."

The leaders of candomblé rituals are drawn from all occupations and sectors of the society. They become ritual leaders and healers because they are believed to have been singled out by the spirits as having the inherent capacity to commune with the spirit world. When leader-healers enter trance and so commune with the spirit world, it is believed that one particular and quite recognizable spirit possesses them and, while they are possessed, speaks and acts through them. Therefore, candomblé leader-healers are believed to be the agents of transmission of the wisdom of the gods during the time they are entranced. Like the *houngans* in voodoo rituals, candomblé leader-healers are assisted by a considerable number of attendants, some of whom have themselves found their calling as messengers of the spirit world, capable of performing some healing activities when possessed by the spirits.

As with voodoo, the pantheon of spirits in candomblé contains both male and female entities and includes the spirits of wise and elderly former slaves of African ancestry. Appeal to those spirits is particularly popular with people beset by familial problems, such as marital infidelity, boyfriends' or girlfriends' unwillingness to commit themselves in a relationship, rejection by partners in intimate relationships, or youth behaving in defiance of parental authority, using street drugs, or being involved in delinquent and criminal behaviors. When possessed by the spirits of former African slaves, candomblé leader-healers assume the characteristic behaviors attributed to the elderly former slaves: sitting on a low stool, puffing constantly on a pipe, and taking frequent swigs from a rum bottle placed beside the stool.

Some spirits are believed to be particularly adept at serving as a medium of communication with deceased relatives and friends. Others are thought to represent the spirits of deceased priests, nuns, or other religious leaders, as well as celebrated past political figures and "national heroes" such as soccer stars and film celebrities.

In order to enter into effective communication with the spirit world, supplicants must prepare themselves for these ritualized encounters by trying to clarify the problem they are experiencing. To do so, they and/or their accompanying family and friends briefly outline the issues of the supplicant's preoccupation to the leader-healer's attendants. In this way, a supplicant is led to the properly designated entranced and spirit-possessed medium, who, with his or her assistant healers, aids the supplicant in praying, contemplating, and ultimately entering the communicative world of the spirits through trance. As this state is achieved, supplicants often become agitated, uncoordinated, and erratic in their movements; swoon or fall to the floor; and/or manifest seizure-like contractions of their bodies. They may also speak in tongues. Some people who are thought to be in particularly intense emotional turmoil may rush wildly around the healing area, writhe vigorously on the floor, or thrash out at the assistant healers and attendants. At such times, the supplicants are given the help and constraint they need to avoid hurting themselves or others participating in the rituals, until they become calm enough to be looked after by their accompanying family and friends. The process of return to their pre-trance personality characteristics occurs over a period of minutes to hours.

It is expected that supplicants and those who accompany them to candomblé rituals will make a contribution of money, clothing, and/or food for the benefit of the leader-healer, his or her assistants and attendants, the upkeep of the ceremonial site, and the needs of the community.

Umbanda. Another form of ritualistic healing that closely parallels the candomblé ritual in Brazil is *umbanda,*

> . . . [an] animistic-spiritistic religion . . . with several million adherents espe-
> cially in the bigger cities. It may be characterized as an extra-ecclesiastic consol-
> idation of popular Catholicism within the vacant forms of ancient Afro-
> Brazilian sects. The central belief is the existence of all sorts of spirits; a central
> task is to give them the opportunity temporarily to take hold of human bodies.
> (Figge 1975, p. 246; see also Brown 1986; Brumana and Martinez 1989)

Umbanda contains many of the same elements found in candomblé—belief in the omnipresence of spirits, possession, and highly dramaturgic and
compelling rituals directed toward relief of a wide variety afflictions.

Conclusions

"In the end is the beginning"—both "psychiatry" and "religion" are institutions developed over the course of cultural evolution to address and provide
some relief for the inevitable problems that occur in the course of family and
social interactions. In that respect, both are important in the maintenance of
health and recovery from illness (including but not confined to psychologi-
cal/psychiatric disorders), as well as in the future avoidance of illness and
other misfortunes of life. Prince (1976) has succinctly summarized what appear to be common elements of a very widespread pattern of symbolic healing, elements represented here in the language of psychiatry but correlatively
echoed in the behavioral aspects of religion:

> . . . the special relationship between the healer and the patient; the shared
> world view; the expectant hope of the patient; naming of the illness, attribution
> of cause, and prescription of treatment by the healer; and the central role of
> suggestion. (p. 115)

The extent to which a given analyst—whether priest/minister/leader,
physician/psychiatrist, or patient—may opt for one conceptual/epistemolog-
ical framework over another is irrelevant. Indeed, many individuals, in quite
diverse cultural settings, combine belief systems rather than differentially
choose one or the other belief system and adhere to it exclusively under all
circumstances. For example, many scientists who are conforming believers in
a religious creed are nonetheless able—through the powerful psychological
principle of compartmentalization—to shift comfortably into the empirical
scientific frame of reference in their work.

The intent of this chapter has been to describe those empirically observable patterns of behavior that are—and in our view must be—considered the primary data from which either kind of conceptualization—religious or scientific—derives. The phenomenological aspects of human behavior do not present with premarked seams for separating out analytic categories; rather, they admit of a variety of interpretations (Watzlawick 1984). In this way,

> "religion," "medicine," and "morality" are frequently found together in the same behavioral act or event . . . . (Hughes 1968, p. 87)

References

American Psychiatric Association: Diagnostic and Statistical Manual of Mental Disorders, 4th Edition. Washington, DC, American Psychiatric Association, 1994

Baker B: The mind-body connection: putting the "faith factor" to work. AARP Bulletin 38(7):20, 1997

Benson H: Timeless Healing: The Power and Biology of Belief. New York, Scribner, 1996

Bourguignon E: World distribution and patterns of possession states, in Trance and Possession States. Edited by Prince R. Montreal, Canada, Proceedings, Second Annual Conference, R. M. Bucke Memorial Society, 1966, pp 3–34

Bourguignon E: Possession and trance in cross-cultural studies of mental health, in Culture-Bound Syndromes, Ethnopsychiatry, and Alternative Therapies. Edited by Lebra WP. Honolulu, HI, University of Hawaii Press, 1976, pp 47–55

Brown DDG: Umbanda: Religion and Politics in Urban Brazil. Ann Arbor, MI, University of Michigan Research Press, 1986

Brumana FG, Martinez EG: Spirits From the Margin: Umbanda in Sao Paulo, A Study in Popular Religion and Social Experience. Uppsala, Sweden, Almqvist & Wiksell International, 1989

Carrese JA, Rhodes LA: Western bioethics on the Navajo reservation: benefit or harm? JAMA 274:826–829, 1995

Condon G: Rx for healing: take 2 aspirin and pray in the morning. Salt Lake Tribune, July 15, 1995, p 1

Crapanzano V: Hamadsha: A Study in Moroccan Ethnopsychiatry. Berkeley, CA, University of California Press, 1973

Crapanzano V: Saints, jnun, and dreams: an essay in Moroccan ethnopsychology. Psychiatry 38:145–159, 1975

Crapanzano V, Garrison V (eds): Case Studies in Spirit Possession. New York, Wiley, 1977

Csordas TJ: The rhetoric of transformation in ritual healing. Cult Med Psychiatry 7:333–375, 1983

Csordas TJ, Kleinman A: The therapeutic process, in Medical Anthropology: Contemporary Theory and Method, Revised Edition. Edited by Sargent CF, Johnson TM. Westport, CT, Praeger, 1996, pp 3–20

Dow J: Universal aspects of symbolic healing: a theoretical synthesis. American Anthropologist 88:56–69, 1986

Faith and healing (special issue). Time, June 24, 1996, pp 58–62

Figge HH: Spirit possession and healing cult among the Brasilian umbanda. Psychother Psychosom 25:246–250, 1975

Frank JD, Frank JB: Persuasion and Healing: A Comparative Study of Psychotherapy, 3rd Edition. Baltimore, MD, Johns Hopkins University Press, 1993

Goodenough WH: Evolution of the human capacity for beliefs. American Anthropologist 92:597–612, 1990

Goodman N: Ways of Worldmaking. Indianapolis, IN, Hackett, 1978

Griffin DR: Introduction: postmodern spirituality and society, in Spirituality and Society: Postmodern Visions. Edited by Griffin DR. Albany, NY, State University of New York Press, 1988, pp 1–31

Harding TW: Traditional healing methods for mental disorders. WHO Chronicle 31:436–440, 1975

Hughes CC: Anthropological fieldnotes from St. Lawrence Island, Alaska (Eskimo), 1955

Hughes CC: Ethnomedicine, in International Encyclopedia of the Social Sciences, Vol 10. Edited by Sills D. New York, Macmillan, 1968, pp 87–92

Kenney MG: Multiple personality and spirit possession. Psychiatry 44:337–358, 1981

Kiev A: Spirit possession in Haiti. Am J Psychiatry 118:133–138, 1961

Kiev A: The psychotherapeutic value of spirit-possession in Haiti, in Trance and Possession States. Edited by Prince R. Montreal, Canada, Proceedings, Second Annual Conference, R. M. Bucke Memorial Society, 1966, pp 143–148

Kiev A: Transcultural Psychiatry. New York, Free Press, 1972

Kluckhohn C, Leighton DC: The Navaho. Cambridge, MA, Harvard University Press, 1948

LaBarre W: They Shall Take Up Serpents: Psychology of the Southern Snake-Handling Cult. Minneapolis, MN, University of Minnesota Press, 1962

Leighton AH, Leighton DC: Elements of psychotherapy in Navaho religion. Psychiatry IV:515–524, 1941

Leighton AH, Leighton DC: The Navaho Door: An Introduction to Navaho Life. Cambridge, MA, Harvard University Press, 1945

Lommel A: Shamanism: The Beginnings of Art. New York, McGraw-Hill, 1967

Lukoff D, Lu F, Turner R: Toward a more culturally sensitive DSM-IV: psychoreligious and psychospiritual problems. J Nerv Ment Dis 180:673–682, 1992

Lukoff D, Lu FG, Turner R: Cultural considerations in the assessment and treatment of religious and spiritual problems. Psychiatr Clin North Am 18:467–485, 1995

Maduro RJ: Hoodoo possession in San Francisco: notes on therapeutic aspects of regression. Ethos 3(3):425–447, 1975

Miller WR, Martin JE: Spirituality and behavioral psychology: toward integration, in Behavior Therapy and Religion: Integrating Spiritual and Behavioral Approaches to Change. Edited by Miller WR, Martin JE. Newbury Park, CA, Sage, 1988, pp 13–23

Mischel W, Mischel F: Psychological aspects of spirit possession. American Anthropologist 60:249–260, 1958

Moerman DE: Physiology and symbols: the anthropological implications of the placebo effect, in The Anthropology of Medicine: From Culture to Method. Edited by Romanucci-Ross L, Moerman DE, Tancredi LR. New York, Praeger, 1983, pp 156–167

Montagu A: Touching: The Human Significance of the Skin. New York, Harper & Row (Perennial Library), 1971

Ness RM, Wintrob RM: The emotional impact of fundamentalist religious participation: an empirical study of intra-group variation. Am J Orthopsychiatry 50:302–315, 1980

Ness RM, Wintrob RM: Folk healing: a description and synthesis. Am J Psychiatry 138:1477–1481, 1981

Northrop FSC: The Meeting of East and West: An Inquiry Concerning World Understanding. New York, Macmillan, 1949

Oesterreich TK: Possession, Demonical and Other, Among Primitive Races, in Antiquity, the Middle Ages, and Modern Times. Secaucus, NJ, University Books, 1966

Omwari MS: The Art and Ritual of Bahian Candomblé. Museum of Cultural History, UCLA, Monograph Series No. 24. Regents of the University of California, 1984

Patel V: Spiritual distress: an indigenous model of nonpsychotic mental illness in primary care in Harare, Zimbabwe. Acta Psychiatr Scand 92:103–107, 1995

Pattison EM: Behavioral psychology and religion: a cosmological analysis, in Behavior Therapy and Religion: Integrating Spiritual and Behavioral Approaches to Change. Edited by Miller WR, Martin JE. Newbury Park, CA, Sage, 1988, pp 171–186

Pattison EM, Wintrob RM: Possession and exorcism in contemporary America. J Operational Psychiatry 12:13–20, 1981

Prince R: Indigenous Yoruba psychiatry, in Magic, Faith, and Healing: Studies in Primitive Psychiatry Today. Edited by Kiev A. London, Free Press, 1964, pp 84–120

Prince R: Psychotherapy as the manipulation of endogenous healing mechanisms: a transcultural survey. Transcultural Psychiatric Research Review 13:115–133, 1976

Reichard G: Distinctive features of Navaho religion. Southwestern Journal of Anthropology 1:199–220, 1945

Rousch W: Herbert Benson: mind-body maverick pushes the envelope. Science 276:357–359, 1997

Seaward BL: Spiritual wellbeing: a health education model. Journal of Health Education 22:166–169, 1991

Seaward BL: Reflections on human spirituality for the worksite. American Journal of Health Promotion 9:165–169, 1995

Sereno R: Obeah, magic, and social structure in the Lesser Antilles. Psychiatry 11:15–32, 1948

Shirokogoroff SM: Psychomental Complex of the Tungus. London, Kegan Paul, Trench, Trubner, 1935

Snow LF: Folk medical beliefs and their implications for care of patients: a review based on studies among black Americans. Ann Intern Med 81:82–96, 1974

Thomson KS: The revival of experiments on prayer. American Scientist 84:532–534, 1996

Tinling DC: Voodoo, rootwork and medicine. Psychosom Med 29:483–491, 1967

Tobin JJ, Friedman J: Spirits, shamans, and nightmare death: survivor stress in a Hmong refugee. Am J Orthopsychiatry 53:439–448, 1983

Turner V: Religious specialists: an anthropological study, in International Encyclopedia of the Social Sciences, Vol 13. Edited by Sills D. New York, Macmillan & Free Press, 1968, pp 437–444

Ventis WL: The relationships between religion and mental health. J Social Issues 51:33–48, 1995

Walsh RN: The Spirit of Shamanism. New York, GP Putnam, 1990

Watzlawick P (ed): The Invented Reality: How Do We Know What We Believe We Know? Contributions to Constructivism. New York, WW Norton, 1984

Wintrob RM: Psychosis in association with possession by genii in Liberia. Psychopathologie Africaine 2:249–258, 1966

Wintrob RM: The influence of others: witchcraft and rootwork as explanations of behavior disturbances. J Nerv Ment Dis 156:318–326, 1973

Wintrob RM: Belief and behavior: cultural factors in the recognition and treatment of mental illness, in Current Perspectives in Cultural Psychiatry. Edited by Foulks E, Wintrob R, Westermeyer J, et al. New York, Spectrum, 1977, pp 103–111

Psychoanalysis and Religion

Current Perspectives

W. W. Meissner, S.J., M.D.

The interface between psychoanalysis and religion has emerged over the years as one of the most fascinating and challenging areas of interaction between a clinical, an empirical, and a scientifically oriented discipline on the one hand and a humanistic, revelatory, and transcendental discipline on the other. The history of this engagement is one of constant struggle to find the common ground of dialogue while remaining respectful and tolerant of the disciplinary constraints and commitments of the other side. The discussion has evolved from Freudian origins, cast in iconoclastic, antitheistic, and agnostic terms, into a heated debate between protagonists and antagonists on both sides, and finally to a more meaningful and constructive dialogue among the engaged participants. Within psychoanalysis, the mind-set has progressed from a vision of analysis as an applied science (by which I mean to suggest that the intent was to apply psychoanalytic analyses to the material of other disciplines, thus bringing the resources of analytic interpretation and understanding to enrich those disciplines) to a more balanced and egalitarian view of the dialogue as an exercise in interdisciplinary study (whereby both disciplines undertake the study of areas of common interest, each seeking to learn from the other and adapting their understanding accordingly). The shift from a somewhat authoritarian application to interdisciplinary collaboration has revolutionized the psychoanalytic study of religion and the religious integration of psychoanalytic insights.

Freud

The history of the dialogue between psychoanalysis and religion has its origins in Freud's reflections on religion. From his earliest animadversions on religion as comparable to obsessional neurosis (1907/1959) and the phylogenetic fantasies expounded in "Totem and Taboo" (1913/1957) to his definitive formulations in "The Future of an Illusion" (1927/1961) and the personal ruminations in "Moses and Monotheism" (1939/1964), Freud's highly prejudicial and rationalistic views laid the foundations for the tenor of the ensuing dialogue. Freud's view was essentially that religion was a form of illusion or even—to the extent that it transcended the data of reality—a mass delusion (Freud 1930/1961).

Freud's approach to religion has been roundly criticized and called into question. In fact, his views met staunch rebuttal almost from the beginning. His longtime friend and admirer, the Zurich Lutheran pastor Oskar Pfister, on Freud's invitation, wrote an extensive rejoinder to "Future," titled "The Illusion of a Future" (Pfister 1928/1993), in which he tallied many of the arguments and observations that have echoed throughout the ensuing debate. Briefly, Pfister argued that Freud had allowed himself to be drawn into a view of religion that was highly selective and prejudicial. His early observations of comparable elements in obsessional neurosis and certain forms of religious behavior had led him to regard these as identical. His selection of religious behaviors seemed limited to a relatively low-level and pathologically tinged aspect of religious practice that did not represent the full range of religious experience and reflection. Moreover, Pfister contended, Freud made the mistake of concluding that the presence of pathological indices in religious thinking meant that the truth-value of religious propositions was not only doubtful but negated. These are all highly questionable assumptions and have been analyzed in detail (Meissner 1984, 1992b). In addition to these conceptual flaws, Freud relied on questionable materials and sources that have proven, over the course of time and with the advancement of research findings, to be suspect or fallacious.

Recent years have seen a surge of scholarly revisions of the Freudian story. It turns out that all is not as it seemed, especially regarding Freud's avowed agnosticism. Opinions vary considerably, from Peter Gay's (1987) effort to sustain Freud's avowed self-characterization as "a godless Jew" (a view more recently reinforced by Rizzuto's [1998] detailed reconstruction) to Vitz's (1988) attempt to baptize him as a crypto-Christian. Other efforts at reevaluation have followed a more moderate course, seeking revision without straying into the wilds of questionable or unsubstantiated speculation (Meissner 1984). Material supportive of this direction has been provided in the scholarly reevaluations of Freud's religious views, generally by Wallace (1977, 1978a, 1978b) and particularly touching on his sense of himself in relation to the faith of his forefathers by Rice (1990) and Yerushalmi (1991).

In the nearly threescore years since Freud's death, the psychoanalytic dialogue regarding religion has progressed far beyond the Freudian thesis. Analytic attitudes and assessments of religion have moved to a position of relative antithesis with respect to Freud's arguments. We can hope that further progress will draw us closer to a meaningful synthesis that will allow the powerful resource of analytic understanding to illumine and enrich our understanding of and engagement in the religious sphere. The purpose of this chapter is to review some of the more salient post-Freudian developments and to bring the debate up to its current status.

In the Shadow of the Master

Even before Freud passed from the scene, the currents of thinking on matters religious had begun to divide and flow into divergent channels. Most noteworthy in this respect was the thinking of Carl Jung. Not long after the disruption of his ambivalent relationship with Freud, Jung began to formulate what would become his characteristic approach to religion—an approach resonant with, if not influenced by, Freud's phylogenetic preoccupations as expressed in "Totem and Taboo" (1913/1957). Although the factors contributing to the rupture of the Freud–Jung relationship were complex and far-reaching, religion was without doubt a salient component. Not only was Jung's personal religious experience tainted by his own psychopathology, but his thinking generally tended toward a preoccupation with the mystical and esoteric. Many of Jung's conceptions about religion were immersed in superstition and the occult, with the result that his ambivalent and ambiguous role in the psychoanalytic movement grew more tenuous and conflictual. Jung became more interested in the numinous than the neurotic.

Whereas Freud's view of religion was essentially reductionistic, regarding religious beliefs as little more than forms of illusory wish-fulfillment, Jung followed a much different path. For him, God was a psychic—and therefore nonphysical—reality whose existence could only be established by psychic means. In Jung's view, such psychic facts were real, but real as psychic and not physical phenomena. Jung never clarified this distinction between psychic reality and actual existence; he was concerned exclusively with "psychic truth." This basically Kantian position—that is, restricting knowledge to psychic appearance and relegating reality to the unknown—served only to prolong the ambiguity between Jung's psychoanalytically derived view and traditional religious convictions. Freud could dispense with God, but for Jung, God was a necessary and inevitable psychic fact. For Jung, the question of God's reality and nature was divorced from the epistemological problem of the relationship between subjective human experience and the objective realm; in contrast, Freud had no other god but truth and insisted on the congruence between subjectivity and objectivity. Jung protested that he was dealing with religion purely as a physician and empirically; he was only interested in evaluating concepts *about* God—about God Himself he had nothing to say. Beyond these antitheses lay the more profound epistemological difference that was at the root of the opposition between Freud and Jung. For Freud, religion was the illusion, science the truth. For Jung, both religion and science were forms of myth, each able to gain only limited access to the true nature of reality, and each in its own way a form of "illusion."

Analysts within the Freudian group, however, quickly took up Freud's critique of religion in an effort to deepen and extend its range of implication. Theodore Reik (1931, 1951), for example, extended the Freudian perspective to aspects of religious dogma, ritual, prayer, and guilt. Other authors, such as Ernst Jones (1951/1974), Sidney Tarachow (1952a, 1952b), and Mortimer Ostow (Ostow and Scharfstein 1954), contributed extensive analyses of religious beliefs and practices, following along essentially Freudian lines.

Reactions

At the same time, a vigorous countercurrent of opinion arose, challenging the basically reductionistic applications of analytic conceptualizations to religious matters. There was, of course, a predictable response from religionists of all persuasions. Some reacted to Freud's atheistic and rationalistic pronouncements in antagonistic and denunciatory terms. Protests and counterarguments came from the Franciscan Peter Dempsey and from Dominicans Victor McNabb and Victor White. Roland Dalbiez (1941) provided a comprehensive critique distinguishing between the value of Freud's views regarding psycho-

dynamics and motivation and the misapprehensions underlying his formulations regarding morality and religious and spiritual matters. Others followed a
more compromising path in an attempt to enter into a potentially fruitful dialogue that could enrich both psychoanalytic and religious approaches (Wolman
1976). Hans Küng (1979/1990) contributed a thoughtful reprise of contra-
Freudian arguments. Further contributions to this line of thinking came from
the French analysts Marie Choisy (1950), the Jesuit Louis Beirnaert (1949,
1950, 1952), and René Laforgue (1948, 1949a, 1949b), to name a few, and
from English-speaking analysts such as Lawrence Kubie (1950), Roy Lee
(1949), and Gregory Zilboorg (1958). These authors accepted the Freudian
critique as having limited validity and sought to separate the potentially useful
insights of Freud's analysis from the biases, distortions, and questionable suppositions of his argument. The hope was that the residue of analytic implication would offer a meaningful basis for a deeper and more fruitful
understanding of religious beliefs and cultic praxis. After all, Freud himself
had left a significant loophole in *Future* when he wrote, regarding protests to
his argument:

> An outcry of this kind will really be disagreeable to me on account of my many
> fellow-workers, some of whom do not by any means share my attitude to the
> problems of religion. . . . In point of fact psychoanalysis is a method of re-
> search, and an impartial instrument, like the infinitesimal calculus, as it
> were. . . . Nothing that I have said here against the truth-value of religions
> needed the support of psycho-analysis; it had been said by others long before
> analysis came into existence. If the application of the psycho-analytic method
> makes it possible to find a new argument against the truths of religion, *tant pis*
> for religion; but defenders of religion will by the same right make use of psy-
> cho-analysis in order to give full value to the affective significance of religious
> doctrines. (Freud 1927/1961, pp. 36–37)

Additional force was lent to the development of psychoanalytic thinking about religion by the argument of Erich Fromm (1950), who clarified
the distinction between relatively immature and pathological forms of
religious expression and more mature expressions of religious belief and
commitment and tried to show that setting up irreconcilable and oppositional alternatives was misleading and fallacious. Further support came
from individuals such as Seward Hiltner (1951), who followed the lead
originally provided by Pfister, arguing that psychoanalysis and religion
shared common interests and urging development of areas of consensus
and exploration of areas of divergence.

Winnicott

It was at this juncture that Donald Winnicott, the English pediatrician-turned-analyst, entered the picture. His seminal contribution provided a breakthrough in analytic thinking about religion. Winnicott's analytic origins lay in the brand of psychoanalysis advanced by Melanie Klein and the British object relations school. He focused on the nature of the interaction between mother and child in the earliest stages of life. The part of Winnicott's thinking that concerns us dealt with the process by which the child achieves its first apprehension of the real world. He described the transition from immersion in the symbiotic orbit of the mother–child unit, through stages of differentiation, and finally to a sense of separate reality. The important step in this process was formation of a "transitional object"—a term referring to the child's attachment to some external real object that became invested with the emotional attachment that had originally belonged to the mother. The new object came to represent and substitute for the mother, thereby facilitating a gradual separation and distancing from the mother. Thus, the child might adopt a teddy bear or a piece of cloth or anything—usually something soft and cuddly—to which he or she would become deeply attached, so that any attempt to remove it from the child met with intense and violent protest.

This transitional object was thus the child's first not-me possession and provided a transition from a realm of complete subjectivity to dawning objectivity. Winnicott (1971) described this phenomenon as involving a transitional space between the mother and the child that became an area of illusion. Essential to the illusion was the fact that it was neither subjective nor objective. In regard to feeding at the breast, for example, Winnicott argued that when the infant's need reached an optimal point, the optimal attunement of the mother caused her to respond by offering the breast. At that point, the infant's experience of the appearance of the breast in conjunction with his need was equivalent to creating the breast his need required. At the same time, the breast preexisted the infant's need and was independent of it. Thus, the breast was simultaneously a subjective creation and an objective reality. At another remove, a teddy bear is both an object created by the child to satisfy his need and an independent object that preexists his need. In this sense, transitional objects are neither exclusively subjective nor exclusively objective—they are both, and it is a mistake to try to separate these perspectives. One does not ask whether the transitional object is real—the question is irrelevant.

Winnicott then extended this analysis of transitional objects to transitional phenomena. In his view, the transitional object is not resolved or repressed in the course of development; rather, it is gradually decathected and loses meaning. It is neither forgotten nor mourned, but rather undergoes diffusion and spreads out over the space separating psychic reality from external reality. This is the field of experience constituting culture, including religion and religious beliefs. The capacity for creating illusory experience thus extends to a range of culturally embedded and meaningful contexts. This area of illusion gradually undergoes degrees of disillusionment, bringing the child more fully into the experience of reality and its demands. This progression in the experience of transitional phenomena is facilitated by the child's emerging capacities for play and for symbolic expression. The stage of playing allows the child the opportunity for free and creative self-expression by which he or she creates an imaginary world of objects and meanings; it also enables him or her to learn and develop capacities and skills leading to more adaptive and constructive emergence into the external world. These processes continue to extend themselves into the realm of cultural activities, where they manifest in forms of artistic expression and the development of cultural meanings and beliefs. A primary locus for such illusory experiences is religion.

The emphasis on "illusion" calls for a clarification of illusion in Freud's vocabulary and illusion in a Winnicottian framework. For Freud, illusions were essentially wish-fulfillments, regardless of their connection with reality. Wishes might find a connection with reality, and to that extent they are realistic. But if wishes have no such connection, they extend beyond the realm of the realistic and reality testing and must be regarded as delusional. Insofar as no evidence could be brought to support the validity of religious beliefs, Freud regarded them as delusional; the fact that no evidence could be provided *against* religious beliefs did not weigh in his perspective. Illusions in the Freudian view are thus pathological and irrational and have no truth-value. In contrast, Winnicott's illusion is both a developmentally necessary bridge between infantile self-absorption and involvement in reality and an essential component of human experience corresponding to profound human needs for symbolic, artistic, and religious meaning and involvement. Human existence, for Winnicott, is not a question of mere matter and satisfaction of biological needs. Humans have higher needs that transcend the merely physical and that lead them to seek meaning and self-expression in the world around them. Without illusion and its correlative creativity, human existence would be bleak indeed. Winnicott's argument again subsumed a point of view articulated originally in Pfister's retort to Freud's *Future*.

Beyond Winnicott

Winnicott's analysis of transitional phenomena and his suggestion that the realm of transitional experience included cultural experience led to a definitive break with the Freudian tradition. Winnicott's original formulation of the transitional object was elaborated and refined so that its developmental role was further defined. The analysis of transitional phenomena then called for further articulation. The first efforts in this direction sought to extend Winnicott's suggestion with respect to both art and religion (Grolnick and Barkin 1978; Meissner 1978; Pruyser 1968, 1983). These early efforts brought a deeper and clearer understanding of the complexity, richness, and scope of transitional phenomena. The concept of transitional phenomena not only lent itself to interesting perspectives on religious aspects of human experience and open fresh paths of investigation, but also laid the ground for more fruitful dialogue between psychoanalysis and religious thinking.

The traditional dialogue had faltered on an almost Cartesian split between subjectivity and objectivity. One might have caricatured Freud's approach in terms of its insistence on the subjectivity of religious experience—that is, Freud regarded religious beliefs and experiences exclusively as products of inner mental life without objective reference. Diametrically opposed was the conviction of religious thinkers that their beliefs had objective reference and truth-value. The twain could not meet as long as the suppositions of the respective sides remained divided. Winnicott made it possible to understand that the subject–object split could be surpassed and supplanted by a way of understanding religious phenomena that declined this dichotomy (Malony and Spilka 1991; Pruyser 1968). Like the transitional object of the child, religious objects could be regarded as transitional, and therefore as neither subjective nor objective. The ecstatic experience of the "presence of God," for example, need not be regarded as merely subjective and hallucinatory but might remain open to objective, even existential, reference. The need to reduce the experience to one or the other was bypassed in the interest of further understanding of the experience as religiously meaningful and psychologically motivated.

The next important step in this progression came with the publication of Rizzuto's study *The Birth of the Living God* (1979). Rizzuto advanced the discussion by focusing the qualities of the transitional realm and transitional phenomena on the God-representation. Among the complex representations that come to populate the child's inner world, the God-representation has a special history and course of development, as well as a special place in the individual's experience of self and the world. The God-representation is compounded out of the odds and ends of representational elements derived from objects in the child's experience—primary among these, of course, are the parents. A basic core component of this integration derives from the mirroring experience or lack of it with the mother; contributions from the side of the father may be added later and amalgamated with reflections of the maternal experience. Development of the God-representation, then, can parallel the development of the self and may come to complement and complete an integrated sense of self.

These formulations gave the transitional sphere in religion a specific focus, and thus contributed to bridging the gap between analytic and religious concepts of God and His meaning in the individual believer's life. Care is required not to mistake Rizzuto's meaning. God is not a transitional object, like Winnicott's teddy bear, in this view. However, the God-representation is transitional in the abovementioned sense that it is internally derived but remains open to external reference—that is, its meaning is both subjective and objective, partaking in the sphere of illusory experience, as Winnicott suggested. God Himself remains transcendent, above human comprehension and grasp; insofar as He is known by limited human minds, He is known both analogously and transitionally.

An additional step along the transitional path was taken in my own (Meissner 1990, 1992c) effort to establish transitional conceptualization as distinct from subjective and objective forms of cognition and as constituting a distinct realm of discourse within which the disparate approaches of psychoanalysis and religious and theological conceptualization could find a common ground. Within this realm, oppositional dichotomies would have less valid and meaningful application. In this perspective, the special qualities of transitional conceptualization allow for statements to be made regarding the psychic origin and implications of religious concepts, embracing the full scope of analytic relevance and significance without at the same time excluding the potential objective reference.

For example, the concept of God can be given a full psychoanalytic rendering and understanding in terms of the formation and implications of the God-representation (Rizzuto 1979) without negating or contradicting the full spectrum of theological conviction and argument regarding the actual existence of God and without necessarily reducing the intelligibility of the concept to limited analytic terms. Or, the psychology of an individual's faith and belief in the real presence of Christ in the Eucharist can be explored and understood without eroding the theological substance and meaning of the sacrament. Thinking in terms of transitional conceptualization can thus provide a bridge between the disparate realms of psychoanalytic and theological or religious discourse and understanding. This mode of thinking substitutes the dialectic of complementary assertion (both/and) for the logic of exclusivity (either/or).

Alternative Currents

This ferment of creative energy has led in several directions that have enriched and extended the dialogue. These various shifts and currents are all more or less contemporaneous with and relatively independent of one another, so that one can consider them as a group without needing to organize them preferentially. One important current was centered in Louvain, Belgium, and found expression in the work of Joseph Nuttin (1962) and later Antoine Vergote (1969, 1988). Largely reflecting the influence of continental phenomenological and existential thought, as well as the linguistic and hermeneutic drift of Jacques Lacan, the thoughtful approach independently fashioned by these thinkers embraced the contributions of psychoanalysis to the understanding of religious experience—particularly when that experience was tinged with the psychopathological—yet declined the push to translate the full range of religious experience in its most meaningful and spiritual dimensions into the reductive terms of instinctual dynamics. In Nuttin's and Vergote's view, the interpenetration of dynamic motivation with spiritual experience could be understood only when the respective contributions of the two approaches were kept in proper perspective and remained within the confines of their respective intelligibilities and explanatory scopes.

Other thinkers have explored the implications of object relations theory and its relevance to an analytic understanding of religious phenomena. Rizzuto's (1979) work can be seen in this perspective, since her interest centered on the formation of the representation of God as an object, a concept that implied certain refinements in thinking about the meaning of object representations and object relations. Further amplifications of this object relations–based inquiry were contributed by McDargh (1983), who, working from the base provided by H. Richard Niebuhr and James Fowler, extended the object relations perspective suggested by Rizzuto and the paradoxical aspects of faith experience underlined by Meissner into the understanding of faith in relation both to the image or representation of God as psychologically conceived and to the actual God of religious belief and conviction. Another contribution along this line came from Moshe Spero (1992), who attempted to bring the resources of object relations theory to the understanding of Judaic belief and practice and to join both of these dimensions into a theory of psychotherapy.

It should not be supposed in this discussion that classical perspectives have fallen into disrepute. From time to time, classical perspectives resurface in a new guise, lending freshness and force to the ongoing discussion. Martin Bergmann's (1992) study of the historical and conceptual impact of sacrifice on religious praxis and belief is a case in point. Bergmann takes up many of the traditional themes but gives them a refreshing twist. He argues that the origins of religion derive from the need to placate the anger of the gods by human sacrifice. In the course of history, this dynamic has undergone increasing repression and sublimation but remains a powerful and active unconscious force in the mind of contemporary man. This religious theme reaches its pinnacle in the sacrificial crucifixion of the Son to the Father so central to Christian belief. Comparison with Freud's analysis reveals that Bergmann's and Freud's arguments touch many of the same bases; however, whereas Freud's argument began with the fictive murder of the primal father, Bergmann traces his thesis through historical sources—a strategy that lends it greater credibility. He also reverses the oedipal dynamic: rather than the murderous rebellion of the son against the father, it is the hostile wish of the father against the son—the "Laius complex"—that becomes the central dynamic.

One of the most significant contributors to the redirection of psychoanalytic thinking about religion was Erik Erikson, not only in his ingenious broadening of the scope of analytic concepts regarding personality development and the formation of identity, but also particularly in his interpretations of Luther (Erikson 1958/1962) and Gandhi (Erikson 1969). Erikson was able to connect the most profoundly spiritual aspects of human experience with fundamental infantile roots and dynamics without entertaining the reductionistic fallacy that had plagued earlier efforts (Meissner 1987; Zock 1990). He wrote:

> But must we call it regression if man thus seeks again the earliest encounters of his trustful past in his efforts to reach a hoped-for and eternal future? Or do religions partake of man's ability, even as he regresses, to recover creatively? At their creative best, religions retrace our earliest inner experiences, giving tangible form to vague evils and reaching back to the earliest individual sources of trust; at the same time, they keep alive the common symbols of integrity distilled by the generations. If this is partial regression, it is a regression which, in retracing firmly established pathways, returns to the present amplified and clarified. (Erikson 1958/1962, p. 264)

It is worth noting that Erikson's revisions paralleled those of Winnicott and that the two are more or less congruent. Erikson gave expression to the dynamics of Winnicott's illusion.

The Current Scene

The framework provided by Erikson's clarifications and by the conceptual directions suggested by Winnicott opens the way to a twofold evolution in the psychoanalytic approach to religious matters. The first has a more practical clinical focus; namely, an improved ability to deal empathically and comprehendingly with the religious difficulties and conflicts presented by our patients—a direction taken with increasing seriousness by contemporary analysts (Meissner 1991) and a project urged repeatedly by Pruyser (see Malony and Spilka 1991). The second has more theoretical interest; that is, it offers the basis for more meaningful dialectical excursions into realms of theological discourse that in the past have seemed excessively alien or prohibitive. A more direct and purposeful engagement between psychoanalytic perspectives and interpretive resources and areas of not only religious experience but also religious belief and theological understanding becomes increasingly possible. The effort is essentially interdisciplinary and requires a scholarly and disciplined approach, either by individuals sufficiently informed and trained in the respective areas or by groups of experts in the relevant disciplines who are open to and capable of truly interdisciplinary work. My own attempts to close the gap between analytic perspectives and areas of theological conceptualization such as grace and the theological virtues of faith and hope (Meissner 1987) are no more than stumbling beginnings in a vast and problematic field of exploration. The risks are high, but the potential yield in fruitful understanding and enrichment of both areas is immense.

Erikson's excursions into psychohistory, and specifically into the psychobiography of religious figures, has met with sometimes stringent and cautionary criticism (Johnson 1977) but has also stimulated further efforts to probe the psychology of significant religious actors on the human stage. Studies of the psychology of Ignatius of Loyola, mystic and founder of the Jesuits (Meissner 1992a) and of his spirituality (Meissner 1999), and of the 19th-century Bengali mystic and Hindu saint Ramakrishna (Kakar 1991), as well as a recent volume on Jewish mysticism (Ostow 1995) come to mind. These studies include an assessment of mystical experience—an area in which our understanding is limited indeed, and one that provides a unique challenge to analytic resources. The complex questions regarding how infantile dynamics can play a role in the most highly spiritual and ecstatic realms of religious achievement remain challenging and problematic. More efforts in this direction can be expected and are certain to provide an important vehicle for exploring the heights and depths—the limits—of religious experience.

Another telling line of thought comes from the hand of Stanley Leavy

(1988), who followed a more personalist and phenomenological bent, embracing a view of both psychoanalysis and religion as concerned with exploring the essential depths of human experience, and therefore as complementary and mutually supportive efforts. He spoke in a more theological tone when he wrote:

> At the heart of the Christian faith is the revelation of the hidden One, the unseen Creator of all that exists—including our minds—who has worked within the evolving fabric of existence since the beginning and made himself known in Jesus. Every bit of fresh understanding that we gain of the created universe is a new evidence of God's unconcealment, as is every new insight into the meaning of Christ's incarnate life. We can never grasp or understand that life in its fullness. Mankind, even in the Christian dispensation, can neither stand nor understand this reality and tries again and again to conceal the redeeming Presence beneath all-too-human vestments, making out of our infinitely loving God a very human creature of power, pride, rage, and riches. I see an illuminating parallel between the psychoanalytical effort to disclose as much as possible of our deepest personal intentions and the ever-renewed Christian effort to show us the God who revealed and continues to reveal himself. (Leavy 1988, p. 56)

This amounts to a poignant credo of the believing psychoanalyst.

Looking Toward the Future

This chapter's survey has touched on many bases but left many others unexplored.[1] I hope, nonetheless, that the general tenor and movement of thinking about psychoanalysis and religion is clear enough. The field has moved from a position of mutual defensiveness and antagonism to one of mutual respect and increasing tolerance of differences of viewpoint and understanding. The debate has given way to a dialogue.

As the dialogue evolves, however, caution is required. The dialogue cannot be meaningful unless the respective intelligibilities and methodologies, both in their potential resourcefulness and in their limitations, are understood and taken into account. Psychoanalysts must be sensitive to the limits of analytic

---

[1] J. W. Jones (1991) has provided a useful overview of perspectives and opinions in this area. Jones' survey is ample but suffers somewhat from the tendency to squeeze thinkers into rigid categories that become arbitrary and that may not correspond to these authors' own views of their work. Another noteworthy contribution from an intersubjectivist perspective has been provided by Spezzano and Gargiulo (1997).

understanding and method. The psychoanalytic perspective is at best limited and partial—it does not and should not attempt to explain everything, and what it explains is only one dimension of a complex and dense reality. By the same token, theologians and students of religion cannot assume that their analyses and interpretations encompass the full meaning and significance of their subject matter. Whatever the dogmatic or theological implications of a given religious belief or formulation, there are additional reverberations concerning the interpenetration of beliefs, values, and dogmatic truths with human intentionalities and motivations. These reverberations are the province not only of theology but also of psychology. The boundaries between psychoanalysis and religion must remain intact if the dialogue is to have meaning without unnecessary confusion or obfuscation.

That these boundaries are easily eroded or transgressed with little advertence is axiomatic. However interesting and useful certain studies may be, erosion of boundaries can give rise to other problems stemming from the failure to keep in mind what belongs to what domain. I would at least question whether the blending of transference and transcendence in J. W. Jones' book (1991), for example, may not reflect this sort of bleeding of the sacred into the secular or vice versa. By the same token, Spero's (1992) treatment of religious concepts in the therapeutic context, by introducing the objective real existing God as a factor in both the God-representation and the process of therapy, may run similar risks. To be clear, there is a difference between saying that God acts on human beings and that this action can have psychological effects, on the one hand, and saying that God's action is an aspect of psychological processes, on the other. The former preserves the integrity of the respective realms of discourse; the latter overrides them, to the confusion of both. In my view, the fault lies in removing the conceptualization from the range of transitional understanding and reducing the respective concepts to either their subjective or their objective terms.

To conclude, the contest continues, and none of the contestants have yet won the prize. There may be prizes enough for all in the long run—each may have a piece of the complex and elusive whole, but only a piece. But we can continue to nibble away, learning from our mistakes and fashioning the tools of discovery as we go.

References

Beirnaert SJ: La dimension du mythique dans la sacramentalisme chrétien. Eranos Jahrbuch 17:255–286, 1949

Beirnaert SJ: La symbolisme ascensionelle dans la liturgie et la mystique chrétiennes. Eranos Jahrbuch 19:41–63, 1950

Beirnaert SJ: L'Eglise et la psychanalyse. Etudes 275:229–237, 1952

Bergmann MS: In the Shadow of Moloch: The Sacrifice of Children and Its Impact on Western Religions. New York, Columbia University Press, 1992

Choisy M: Psychanalyse et Catholicisme. Paris, L'Arche, 1950

Dalbiez R: Psychoanalytical Method and the Doctrine of Freud. London, Longmans, Green and Company, 1941

Erikson EH: Young Man Luther: A Study in Psychoanalysis and History (1958). New York, WW Norton, 1962

Erikson EH: Gandhi's Truth: On the Origins of Militant Nonviolence. New York, WW Norton, 1969

Freud S: Obsessive actions and religious practices (1907), in The Standard Edition of the Complete Psychological Works of Sigmund Freud, Vol 9. Translated and edited by Strachey J. London, Hogarth, 1959, pp 115–127

Freud S: Totem and taboo (1913), in The Standard Edition of the Complete Psychological Works of Sigmund Freud, Vol 13. Translated and edited by Strachey J. London, Hogarth, 1957, pp vii–162

Freud S: The future of an illusion (1927), in The Standard Edition of the Complete Psychological Works of Sigmund Freud, Vol 21. Translated and edited by Strachey J. London, Hogarth, 1961, pp 1–56

Freud S: Civilization and its discontents (1930), in The Standard Edition of the Complete Psychological Works of Sigmund Freud, Vol 21. Translated and edited by Strachey J. London, Hogarth, 1961, pp 59–145

Freud S: Moses and monotheism (1939), in The Standard Edition of the Complete Psychological Works of Sigmund Freud, Vol 23. Translated and edited by Strachey J. London, Hogarth, 1964, pp 1–137

Fromm E: Psychoanalysis and Religion. New Haven, CT, Yale University Press, 1950

Gay P: A Godless Jew: Freud, Atheism, and the Making of Psychoanalysis. New Haven, CT, Yale University Press, 1987

Grolnick SA, Barkin L (eds): Between Fantasy and Reality: Transitional Objects and Phenomena. New York, Jason Aronson, 1978

Hiltner S: Self-Understanding Through Psychology and Religion. New York, Scribner, 1951

Johnson RA (ed): Psychohistory and Religion: The Case of Young Man Luther. Philadelphia, PA, Fortress Press, 1977

Jones E: Psycho-myth, Psycho-history: Essays in Applied Psychoanalysis (1951), Vol 2. New York, Hillstone, 1974

Jones JW: Contemporary Psychoanalysis and Religion: Transference and Transcendence. New Haven, CT, Yale University Press, 1991

Kakar S: The Analyst and the Mystic: Psychoanalytic Reflections on Religion and Mysticism. Chicago, IL, University of Chicago Press, 1991

Kubie LS: Psychoanalysis and healing by faith. Pastoral Psychol 1:13–18, 1950

Küng H: Freud and the Problem of God (1979). New Haven, CT, Yale University Press, 1990

Laforgue R: Réflexions d'un psychanalyste. Psyché 3:752–754, 1948

Laforgue R: Au delà du scientisme, I: Freud et le monotheisme. Psyché 4:2–29, 1949a

Laforgue R: Au delà du scientisme, II: psychologie du mérite et del la grâce. Psyché 4:30–49, 1949b

Leavy SA: In the Image of God: A Psychoanalyst's View. New Haven, CT, Yale University Press, 1988

Lee RS: Freud and Christianity. New York, AA Wyn, 1949

Malony HN, Spilka B (eds): Religion in Psychodynamic Perspective: The Contributions of Paul W. Pruyser. New York, Oxford University Press, 1991

McDargh J: Psychoanalytic Object Relations Theory and the Study of Religion: On Faith and the Imaging of God. Lanham, MD, University Press of America, 1983

Meissner WW: Psychoanalytic aspects of religious experience. Ann Psychoanal 6:103–141, 1978

Meissner WW: Psychoanalysis and Religious Experience. New Haven, CT, Yale University Press, 1984

Meissner WW: Life and Faith: Psychological Perspectives on Religious Experience. Washington, DC, Georgetown University Press, 1987

Meissner WW: The role of transitional conceptualization in religious thought, in Psychoanalysis and Religion. Edited by Smith JH, Handelman SA. Baltimore, MD, Johns Hopkins University Press, 1990, pp 95–116

Meissner WW: The phenomenology of religious psychopathology. Bull Menninger Clin 55:281–298, 1991

Meissner WW: Ignatius of Loyola: The Psychology of a Saint. New Haven, CT, Yale University Press, 1992a

Meissner WW: The pathology of belief systems. Psychoanalysis Contemp Thought 15:99–128, 1992b

Meissner WW: Religious thinking as transitional conceptualization. Psychoanal Rev 79:175–196, 1992c

Meissner WW: To the Greater Glory—A Psychological Study of Ignatian Spirituality (Marquette Studies in Theology, No. 16). Milwaukee, WI, Marquette University Press, 1999

Nuttin J: Psychoanalysis and Personality: A Dynamic Theory of Normal Personality. New York, New American Library, 1962

Ostow M (ed): Ultimate Intimacy: The Psychodynamics of Jewish Mysticism. Madison, CT, International Universities Press, 1995

Ostow M, Scharfstein B-A: The Need to Believe: The Psychology of Religion. New York, International Universities Press, 1954

Pfister O: The illusion of a future: a friendly disagreement with Prof. Sigmund Freud (with an introduction by P. Roazen) (1928). International Journal of Psychoanalysis 74:557–579, 1993

Pruyser PW: A Dynamic Psychology of Religion. New York, Harper & Row, 1968

Pruyser PW: The Play of the Imagination. New York, International Universities Press, 1983

Reik T: Ritual: Psychoanalytic Studies. London, Hogarth, 1931

Reik T: Dogma and Compulsion: Psychoanalytic Studies of Religion and Myths. New York, International Universities Press, 1951

Rice E: Freud and Moses: The Long Journey Home. Albany, NY, State University of New York Press, 1990

Rizzuto A-M: The Birth of the Living God. Chicago, IL, University of Chicago Press, 1979

Rizzuto A-M: Why Did Freud Reject God? A Psychodynamic Interpretation. New Haven, CT, Yale University Press, 1998

Spero MH: Religious Objects as Psychological Structures: A Critical Integration of Object Relations Theory, Psychotherapy, and Judaism. Chicago, IL, University of Chicago Press, 1992

Spezzano C, Gargiulo GJ (eds): Soul on the Couch : Spirituality, Religion, and Morality in Contemporary Psychoanalysis (Relational Perspectives Book Series, Vol 7). Hillsdale, NJ, Analytic Press, 1997

Tarachow S: Applied psychoanalysis, II: religion. Ann Survey Psychoanalysis 1:312–317, 1952a

Tarachow S: Applied psychoanalysis, II: religion and mythology. Ann Survey Psychoanalysis 3:494–510, 1952b

Vergote A: The Religious Man: A Psychological Study of Religious Attitudes. Dayton, OH, Pflaum Press, 1969

Vergote A: Guilt and Desire: Religious Attitudes and Their Pathological Derivatives. New Haven, CT, Yale University Press, 1988

Vitz PC: Sigmund Freud's Christian Unconscious. New York, Guilford, 1988

Wallace ER: The psychodynamic determinants of "Moses and Monotheism." Psychiatry 40:79–87, 1977

Wallace ER: Freud's father conflict: the history of a dynamic. Psychiatry 41:33–56, 1978a

Wallace ER: Freud's mysticism and its psychodynamic determinants. Bull Menninger Clin 42:203–222, 1978b

Winnicott DW: Playing and Reality. New York, Basic Books, 1971

Wolman BB (ed): Psychoanalysis and Catholicism. New York, Gardner, 1976

Yerushalmi YH: Freud's Moses: Judaism Terminable and Interminable. New Haven, CT, Yale University Press, 1991

Zilboorg G: Freud and Religion. Westminster, MD, Newman, 1958

Zock H: A Psychology of Ultimate Concern: Erik H. Erikson's Contribution to the Psychology of Religion (International Series in the Psychology of Religion). Atlanta, GA, Editions Rodopi, 1990

✧ CHAPTER 4 ✧

A Psychological Perspective on Cults

Marc Galanter, M.D.

Contemporary cults exercise intense group influence and can have a major impact on their members' behavior. By drawing on empirical research and descriptive accounts of recent cult activity, this chapter describes a generic model for such cohesive, intensely ideological groups and examines the psychological forces they draw on. In particular, I will describe the characteristics of these phenomena by recourse to the model of the *charismatic group*. The model of the charismatic group (Galanter 1978, 1989b) can be used generically to describe contemporary cults and zealous self-help movements. Such a group is characterized by: 1) a high level of social cohesiveness, 2) an intensely held belief system, and 3) a profound influence on its members' behavior. It is "charismatic" because of the commitment of members to a fervently espoused, transcendent goal; indeed, this goal is frequently articulated by a charismatic leader or ascribed to the progenitor of the group. As we shall see, charismatic groups can relieve certain symptoms associated with psychopathology, although they can precipitate psychiatric symptoms as well.

Among zealous groups, the concept of a *cult* is more specifically religious. It connotes deviancy from established belief and often transcendental experiences (Nelson 1972). Some contemporary religious cults have been called New Religious Movements by writers who are attentive to their potential for finding a place in the religious mainstream (Galanter 1989a; Needleman and

Baker 1978). Those cultic groups that conform to the definition of the charismatic group will be discussed here.

A charismatic group, or cult with a religious orientation, differs from conventional religious groups. It elicits a singular and intense commitment from its members and maintains control over their behavior. It is typically removed from the cultural mainstream and promotes a relatively isolated culture and lifestyle. Conventional religious groups in our American society, on the other hand, do elicit fealty and regularity of practice, but they reflect the multiple ties—often competing—of a pluralistic society; in addition, the behavioral norms they espouse are loosely applied. Conventional religious groups are melded into the body politic.

A Historical Perspective on the Conversion Experience

William James (1902/1929; also see Chapter 8 in this volume) wrote about religious conversion as a process through which an individual, "divided and consciously wrong, inferior and unhappy" becomes "unified and consciously right, superior and happy" as a consequence of achieving a hold on his or her religious reality. It may otherwise be described as a process by which a person comes to adopt an all-pervasive worldview.

Transcendental or mystical experiences are often important in the conversion process, as noted by both James (1902/1929) and Freud (1921/1955). The importance of transcendental experiences in conflict resolution, even to the point of precipitating acute hallucinatory episodes in both nonpsychotic (Jacobsen 1964; Sterba 1968) and psychotic (Sedman and Hopkinson 1966) individuals, has also been emphasized. These experiences are also integral to continuing group membership (Buckley and Galanter 1979; Galanter and Buckley 1978) for many members of charismatic sects.

Psychological Forces in the Group

In order to understand how charismatic groups can profoundly shape the thinking and behavior of their members, we will consider the psychological forces they employ, which are brought to bear on the preexisting disposition and psychology of recruits. One of these forces, *group cohesiveness*, is defined as the result of all the forces that act on members to keep them engaged in a group (Cartwright and Zander 1962). When cohesiveness is strong, participants work to sustain the commitment of their fellow members, to protect them from threat, and to ensure the safety of shared resources. This can lead, as Pattison and others have pointed out, to members' experiencing psycho-therapeutic benefit (Galanter 1989b; Kilbourne and Richardson 1984; Levine 1983; Pattison 1977).

The impact of group cohesiveness on the psychological status of members was evident in a study my colleagues and I conducted of a contemporary charismatic sect, the Divine Light Mission (Galanter 1978; Galanter and Buckley 1978). Young adult members of the group reported appreciable psychiatric problems before joining. For example, 30% had sought professional help, and 9% had been hospitalized for emotional disorders. Furthermore, members' self-reports reflected a considerable relief in neurotic distress after they affiliated with the group. Their responses also demonstrated an intense social cohesiveness with the group that was highly correlated with the degree of symptom relief evidenced by individual members.

Shared belief, a second force operative in the charismatic group, was evident in studies conducted by myself and my associates on the psychological well-being of long-standing Unification Church members (Galanter et al. 1979). Measures of social cohesiveness and religious belief accounted for a large portion of the variance in contemporaneous well-being (i.e., their state at that time), and items that measured religious belief were the highest-ranking predictors of well-being. This finding suggests the additional role of belief as a motivating force in charismatic groups. It also demonstrates the importance of healers and their patients having a shared set of beliefs about illness and treatment. Kleinman and Gale (1982) found this "explanatory model" to be an important component of treatment effectiveness in their cross-cultural studies of shamanistic healing.

Altered consciousness is another force operating in the charismatic group. This phenomenon is frequently described by contemporary cult members (Galanter 1989b; Needleman and Baker 1978) and is typically elicited in an intense group experience. As has been pointed out in relation to religious conversion (Proudfoot and Shaver 1976), such an experience can serve as the basis upon which converts come to attribute a new worldview of meaning to their lives. In the Divine Light Mission and Unification Church samples (Galanter and Buckley 1978; Galanter et al. 1979), for example, my colleagues and I found experiences of altered consciousness to be significantly correlated with the improved affective status experienced by members upon conversion.

In the charismatic group, these forces operate to compel *behavioral conformity* and modulate affect, in the absence of overt coercion. In order to understand this process of social control, it is useful to contrast it with the influence effected in brainwashing. Brainwashing was described by Lifton

(1961) among prisoners of the Korean War who were forcibly confined by the Communist Chinese. In both brainwashing scenarios and charismatic groups, those directing the process maintain control over the "context of communication" in order to prevent expression of perspectives contrary to their own. In the brainwashing setting, however, participants are imprisoned and physically coerced. Members of charismatic groups are not; instead, the psychological forces described above—altered consciousness, shared beliefs, and group cohesiveness—cause new meaning and values to be attributed to members' experience by means of social reinforcement of compliance.

How does this reinforcement take place? Findings on the role of these forces suggest the operation of a "relief effect" (Galanter 1978, 1989b; Kilbourne and Richardson 1984; Wenegrat 1989) in the psychiatric impact of charismatic groups. That is to say, a relief in emotional distress is experienced by both new recruits and long-term members when they feel more closely affiliated with the group, whereas a decline in affiliative feelings can result in greater distress. Such an effect, sociobiologically grounded (Galanter 1978) and mediated by the social context, can serve as an operant reinforcer for regulating behavior (Ferster 1958). When a member acts in accordance with the group's expectations, he or she receives positive reinforcement in the form of enhanced well-being; when the member rejects the group's behavioral norms, he or she experiences the negative reinforcement of increased distress. This reinforcement effect also serves to increase the likelihood of the member's maintaining affiliation with the group and complying with its expectations for behavior. Operant conditioning in charismatic groups takes place both informally and in structured rituals.

Because operant reinforcement of approved behaviors can both bring members into compliance with the group and restructure their perceptions of the world around them, such reinforcement can also serve as the basis for a remission in a recruit's pathological perceptions. The enhanced well-being inherent in the affiliation process can then contribute to the relief of major psychopathology, as illustrated by the following case history:

Jim, a 24-year-old technician with no history of psychiatric illness, became increasingly withdrawn over the course of a year after beginning to smoke marijuana. After concluding that his co-workers were conspiring to have him arrested for drug possession, he moved into a secluded rural setting, where he subsequently came to believe that his "soul was moving out" of him and that he saw flying saucers nearby. Soon he felt he was going out of his mind. It was at this point that he encountered members of an Eastern cultic group, who invited him to spend time at their communal residence. After 2 months of meditation and daily attendance at the group's religious services, Jim was no longer anxious or delusional, reporting that he was "at peace with himself." A year later, he had had no recurrence in symptoms and was still involved in the group's activities.

The intense cohesiveness of the charismatic group, in combination with its ability to influence members' beliefs, can yield relief of psychopathology. However, this cohesiveness can also generate psychiatric syndromes, particularly when an individual becomes alienated from a cohesive group but still accepts its belief system. The potent impact of such estrangement, even to the point of inducing psychotic symptoms, is illustrated below:

> Barry, a 16-year-old member of a family belonging to a neo-Christian cult, was admitted to the hospital because he was hearing voices. Both the patient and his collaterals reported that he had never experienced psychiatric difficulties until he was caught smoking marijuana by fellow cult members; the members had then insisted that he was tainted by the Devil because he had violated the group's religious injunction. On the heels of this experience, the youth became alienated and ran off to stay at the home of a relative not affiliated with the cult. Over the course of a month, he became increasingly guilt-ridden and anxious about having left the group and then began to hallucinate the voice of the Devil telling him he had betrayed the cult. His symptoms remitted over the course of a 1-month hospitalization during which he received supportive milieu treatment only.

The Psychiatric Impact of Joining a Charismatic Group

Individual members of contemporary charismatic groups generally state that joining the group has had a positive effect on their psychological state. Interviewers describe reports of new strength and "spiritual resources" as well as reduced "self-hatred" (Nicholi 1974). Increased feelings of calm and happiness and a capacity for better relationships are also noted (Levine and Salter 1976; Wilson 1972). In one series of controlled studies, my associates and I (Galanter 1980, 1981; Galanter and Buckley 1978; Galanter et al. 1979) measured the psychological impact of conversion to the Divine Light Mission and the Unification Church. Structured self-reports of representative samples of members of these groups indicated considerable enhancement of emotional state (the "relief effect") upon joining; this improved state was maintained over the course of long-term membership (2–3 years).

It is interesting, however, that despite the reported improvement, long-term members' scores on the psychological well-being portion of the

General Well-Being Schedule (Dupuy 1973) were slightly below those of an age- and sex-matched sample from the general population. This result was compatible with our finding of even lower scores on psychological well-being for a representative sample of nonmembers who registered for the sects' workshops before joining (Galanter 1980). Members' current levels of psychological well-being were correlated with the intensity of both their social affiliation with other members and their espousal of the group's ideology, indicating that charismatic group members may have an inherent tendency to sustain their affiliation with the group in order to maintain their enhanced emotional state. I have proposed (Galanter 1978, 1981) that humans may possess a biologically grounded propensity to coalesce into such groups, particularly when ties to other sources of affiliation are weakened.

The impact of group forces is felt at each stage of membership in a charismatic group, beginning with induction and continuing through stabilization and departure. A description of the course of membership in the Unification Church will illustrate the operation of these psychological forces. One recruitment format used by the Unification Church is the structured workshop series. In studying this recruitment setting (Galanter 1980), I found that a sizable portion of participants (29%) agreed to stay beyond the weekend for which they were initially invited, and that 9% joined after a full 3-week experience. Analysis of self-report data revealed that workshop participants who stayed beyond the first weekend—even those who did not go on to join—became highly involved in the group process. This occurred both on the level of social cohesiveness and in terms of accepting the group's creed. Compared with workshop participants who did not become members of the church, those who eventually joined were experiencing greater psychological distress before the workshops and had fewer cohesive ties to friends and family outside the group. This finding suggests that individuals who demonstrate even moderate interest in a charismatic group can easily become engaged on an interpersonal and a cognitive level. Long-term engagement, however, may require the fertile soil of psychological distress and alienation.

Group Operation

Once a person joins a charismatic group, his or her behavior is typically subject to the group's control. This control was evident in the marked decline in heavy drug and alcohol use effected by the Unification Church in its recruits and continued with long-term members (Galanter et al. 1979). It was also illustrated in the Unification Church engagement (Galanter 1983a) and marriage rituals (Galanter 1986), since the norms involved in these rituals deviate greatly from those of the American middle class. For example, Reverend Sun Myung Moon himself selected the mates for almost all Church members. A large majority of Unification Church fiancés (87%) reported that they felt no preference at all for any particular individual at the time Moon chose their mate for them, reflecting their compliance on a cognitive level. The affective impact of the aforementioned relief effect was evident in the distress associated with noncompliance; those contemplating severing their engagement were the most severely depressed subgroup of members.

Furthermore, on a 3-year follow-up of the engaged members, despite the remarkably unorthodox nature of the cult's marriage customs, almost all (95%) were still active in the Unification Church and were married to fellow Church members (88%). Members' commitment could be understood by recourse to the model of a "pincer": On the one hand, the Church, like other charismatic groups, created distress by ordering unusual behaviors. On the other, it provided relief when members complied and maintained their commitment to the group.

Members' commitment to a charismatic group is remarkably persistent, even after leaving the group. For example, 3 years after their departure from the Unification Church, ex-members, although typically well adjusted in the general community, still maintained a considerable fidelity toward the group (Galanter 1983b). A sizable majority still cared strongly for the members they knew best and reported that they "got some positive things" out of their involvement with the group. This fidelity is evidence of the potential that a charismatic group has for continuing influence, even after a member departs, as we shall see among self-help groups that operate along similar lines.

To understand why charismatic groups elicit certain puzzling behaviors in their members, it is useful to consider how such groups operate as social systems. As members become part of the social system of the group, they become entrained in the system's need to ensure its own stability. The seemingly pathological behavior of individuals may be no more than responses induced by the group to protect its integrity.

Large-Group Psychology and Psychiatric Assessment: A Formulation

Some characteristics of an open system may relate to our knowledge of charismatic groups. Open systems are characterized by boundary control (Baker 1970; Miller and Rice 1967), by means of which the potential components of the system (people and beliefs, in this case) are either defined as part of the system or kept outside it. In the charismatic group, this boundary control is particularly important because of conflicts between the group's perspectives and those of the general population. A group's ideology does serve as a cognitive basis for the group's boundary control function—to differentiate the group's own members from nonmembers.

Boundary control, like functions of the open system, may help to explain puzzling behaviors observed among members of charismatic large groups. For example, some observers of these groups (Clark 1979; Singer 1978) have described the glazed and withdrawn look of certain sect members. This syndrome may meet criteria for the diagnosis of a dissociative reaction. This diagnosis may apply to "trancelike states" in persons who have been subjected to periods of "intensive coercive persuasion." Although this response may appear pathological when observed in a given individual, it may be quite adaptive for sustaining membership in the group. It may facilitate the members' avoidance of influence from outsiders and can thus be understood as a component of the group's boundary control function, evinced as a demand characteristic of the group. Although such responses may be engendered through membership in the group, they may emerge only in settings that threaten the group's integrity. Thus, an observer who is perceived as antagonistic to the group would be more likely to report this response than one who is not.

For charismatic groups, boundary control is facilitated by the development of the group's distinctive character, whether in dress, custom, or ideology. It is also ensured if the group fosters distrust of outsiders and their beliefs. For example, members have been reported to experience relief of neurotic distress upon joining a group (Galanter 1978, 1981; Galanter et al. 1979). When variables related to social cohesiveness were examined to ascertain which of them were correlated with this relief (Galanter 1978), suspiciousness toward outsiders showed the highest correlation, exceeding even positive feelings toward one's fellow group members. This finding may help to explain the ease with which a defensive "paranoia" may emerge among certain sect members who are pressed by family or strangers to give up their ties to the group. In certain instances, this response may even meet criteria for a shared paranoid disorder—that is, it may be characterized by what seems to be persistent delusional thinking regarding outsiders, in the absence of other psychotic symptoms, and may be engendered by close association with others who have similar "delusions" (i.e., other members). Such shared beliefs—particularly when paranoid in orientation—may serve as the basis for the highly deviant actions undertaken by some groups.

An Illustrative Encounter

Events in Waco, Texas, in 1993 illustrate some important aspects of the psychology of charismatic groups. Altogether, over 100 lives were lost in a confrontation between the United States government and a small cultic offshoot of the Seventh-Day Adventists. Beyond that, however, the episode left open the issue of the credibility of the American justice system for a sizable portion of the population.

Federal involvement with the cultic group began with an initial raid on Ranch Apocalypse, the compound where the members were housed, after reports indicating that the group had accumulated a large cache of weaponry. An initial assault left four federal agents and six cult members dead. A day later, military vehicles were brought in to surround the complex, after which David Koresh, the group's leader, released 10 children. Shortly thereafter, some members of the group left the compound and were arrested, and federal agents reported that Koresh had pledged to surrender after he received an appropriate message from God. A standoff ensued, and after 3 weeks federal agents began what they considered to be a psychological intervention, blaring rock music and Tibetan chants over loudspeakers. Meanwhile, Koresh offered repeated explanations as to when he would respond to requests to leave relative to his divine contacts. On day 51 of the standoff, tanks were used to break through the walls of the compound, firing tear gas inside in an attempt to flush out the cult members, and fires soon broke out, later alleged to be set by the members themselves. This led to a conflagration and to the deaths of Koresh and 80 of his followers.

How did this cultic group devolve into a tragedy of mass suicide? The group was founded in the 1930s as an offshoot of the Seventh-Day Adventist Church and was led by a zealot who believed that the return of Christ was imminent. This provided the religious underpinnings for a belief system that was well established by the time the young Vernon Howell, who later changed his name to David Koresh, arrived at the sect's Waco site in the late 1970s. This long-standing set of beliefs lent weight and credibility to the deviant perspective that Koresh applied to the group's ethos.

Howell acquired the mantle of charisma and won control over the membership by gaining the support and sexual favors of an elderly woman who had been married to the group's recently deceased leader. He later left the group to travel to Israel with the messianic mission of converting the Jews there, and returned to find that the son of the previous leader had taken over the compound. Koresh then undertook an armed guerrilla-like attack on the compound that resulted in an exchange of gunfire. He and seven members of his team were indicted on charges of attempted murder, but their trial ended in a hung jury. All this undoubtedly left the issue of armed assault on the compound prominent in Koresh's thinking, later feeding into his paranoia and leading him to stockpile arms.

What was the role of the group's *beliefs* in the course of these events? Consensual and strongly held beliefs are essential to the integrity of a charismatic group, and Koresh drew on both the millenarian vision of the Adventists (i.e., the belief in messianic arrival) and the American cultural acceptance of bearing arms in his subsequent operation. He employed the concept of active communication with God in his belief system to meet his own purposes. Indeed, when his compound was later surrounded by federal authorities, he presented them with a "letter from God" signed "Yahweh Koresh," and said, "I am your God and you will bow under my feet." By the time this was written, close to the end of the standoff, Koresh had likely slipped into a more gravely deluded state.

As previously noted, *boundary control* is a central issue for the charismatic group. This mechanism is necessary for maintaining the security of the group's ideological base, preserving the integrity of its membership, and protecting the group from outside incursions. This aspect of the group contributed to the siege mentality promoted by Koresh, his acquisition of armaments, and construction of the group's fortress-like residence. It also allowed him to assert an increasing degree of control over the members. Attempts by federal agents to undermine the group's integrity by assaulting the compound with loud noises only bolstered the intensity of the members' commitment to self-defense.

Koresh's role also illustrates the remarkable degree of *behavioral control* seen in such groups. As described earlier in this chapter, compliance with the leader's expectations is promoted by a system of operant reinforcement (the relief effect) in which members' affective status becomes entwined with their degree of commitment in the group. This ability to elicit compliance provided a basis for Koresh to take many of the women in the group as sexual partners who bore him children, while other men and women in the cult were subjected to celibacy. Individuals and couples who could not comply with this demand had long before left the group by the time the confrontation with outside authorities had begun. This left a distillate of the most committed in the compound, with little likelihood of anyone voicing dissent relative to Koresh's views.

With the establishment of new social controls and the introduction of socially deviant values, *conventional norms* were abrogated. A new, strongly held moral system now applied. The collapse of conventional norms was illustrated by the abuse of children. Koresh often beat the boys and engaged girls in sexual activity when they were as young as 10 years old.

Along with the collapse of conventional behavioral norms, the trappings of *psychological stability* were lost to Koresh as typically happens with cult leaders, such as Jim Jones in Guyana. The adulation of his followers does much to induce such grandiosity. And with this collapse comes the loss of a perspective within the leader that would allow for reasoned judgment and a respect for human life. Even before his confrontation with the government, Koresh displayed a grandiosity in his designs for worldwide religious leadership.

As with the other recent cataclysmic decline into mass suicide in Jonestown, the leader of the Davidians needed to avoid the intrusion of an outside perspective into the domain of his cult, and this goal came to predominate over an instinctive inclination to protect his own life and the lives of his followers. As in the psychology of martyrdom for worthwhile causes, such a decision can lead to the demise of the whole group on issues of "principle." For some members of the Waco cult, this fate was accepted in a voluntary manner, and indeed one member of the group had to be restrained by authorities as she attempted to run back into the burning compound. For others, trapped in the midst of the disaster, any attempt to escape would have been impossible.

Federal authorities learned a lesson from the loss of life in Waco as well as from the paranoia generated in right-wing groups by their fear of comparable assault by the central government. A tactic of waiting and watching without provoking a group's need for boundary control, and without adding to the paranoia of a group's leader, has come to be seen as the wiser policy in dealing with such confrontations.

Conclusions

To summarize, in this chapter I have reviewed operational definitions for charismatic groups and cults and have examined the psychological forces that operate to sustain them. We then considered some examples of the impact of this psychology on both individual and group behavior, and examined the way people are inducted into the charismatic group and become integrated into its social system. The behavioral deviancy produced by these groups was considered in the example of the Branch Davidian cult. Although charismatic groups like that one may have a negative, even tragic, impact on their members, the psychological forces that underlie them are inherently value free, so that benevolent outcomes may be experienced in some other zealous groups.

References

Baker F: General systems theory, research, and medical care, in Systems and Medical Care. Edited by Sheldon A, Baker F, McLaughlin CP. Cambridge, MA, MIT Press, 1970, pp 1–26

Buckley P, Galanter M: Mystical experience, spiritual knowledge and a contemporary ecstatic religion. Br J Med Psychol 52:281–289, 1979

Cartwright D, Zander A (eds): Group Dynamics: Research and Theory. Evanston, IL, Row, Peterson, 1962

Clark JG Jr: Cults. JAMA 242:279–281, 1979

Dupuy H: Current health and nutrition examination survey (psychological section), in Proceedings of the Public Health Conference on Records and Statistics—1972 (DHEW Publication 74-1214). Rockville, MD, DHEW, 1973

Ferster CB: Control of behavior in chimpanzees and pigeons by time out from positive reenforcement. Psychol Monogr 461, 1958

Freud S: Group psychology and the analysis of the ego (1921), in The Standard Edition of the Complete Psychological Works of Sigmund Freud, Vol 18. Translated and edited by Strachey J. London, Hogarth, 1955, pp 65–143

Galanter M: The "relief effect": a sociobiological model for neurotic distress and large-group therapy. Am J Psychiatry 135:588–591, 1978

Galanter M: Psychological induction into the large-group: findings from a modern religious sect. Am J Psychiatry 137:1574–1579, 1980

Galanter M: Sociobiology and informal social controls of drinking. J Stud Alcohol 42:64–79, 1981

Galanter M: Engaged members of the Unification Church. Arch Gen Psychiatry 40:1197–1202, 1983a

Galanter M: Unification Church ("Moonie") dropouts: psychological readjustment after leaving a charismatic religious group. Am J Psychiatry 140:984–988, 1983b

Galanter M: Moonies get married: a psychiatric follow-up study of a charismatic religious sect. Am J Psychiatry 143:1245–1249, 1986

Galanter M (ed): Cults and New Religious Movements: A Report of the American Psychiatric Association. Washington, DC, American Psychiatric Press, 1989a

Galanter M: Cults: Faith, Healing and Coercion. New York, Oxford University Press, 1989b

Galanter M, Buckley P: Evangelical religion and meditation: psychotherapeutic effects. J Nerv Ment Dis 166:685–691, 1978

Galanter M, Rabkin R, Rabkin J, et al: The "Moonies": a psychological study. Am J Psychiatry 136:165–170, 1979

Jacobsen E: The Self and the Object World. New York, International Universities Press, 1964

James W: The Varieties of Religious Experience (1902). New York, Modern Library, 1929

Kilbourne B, Richardson JT: Psychotherapy and new religions in a pluralistic society. Am Psychol 39:237–251, 1984

Kleinman A, Gale JG: Patients treated by physicians and folk healers: a comparative outcome study in Taiwan. Cult Med Psychiatry 6:405–423, 1982

Levine S: Alienated Jewish youth and religious seminaries, in Psychodynamic Perspectives on Religion, Sect, and Cult. Edited by Halperin DA. Boston, MA, John Wright PSG, 1983

Levine SV, Salter NE: Youth and contemporary religious movements: psychological findings. Canadian Psychiatric Association Journal 21:411–420, 1976

Lifton RJ: Thought Reform and the Psychology of Totalism. New York, WW Norton, 1961

Miller EJ, Rice AK: Systems of Organization. London, Tavistock, 1967

Needleman J, Baker G (eds): Understanding New Religions. New York, Seabury Press, 1978

Nelson GK: The membership of a cult: the Spiritualists National Union (letter). Review of Religious Research 170:13, 1972

Nicholi AM II: A new dimension of the youth culture. Am J Psychiatry 131:396–401, 1974

Pattison M: A theoretical-empirical base for social systems therapy, in Current Perspectives in Cultural Psychiatry. New York, Tavistock, 1977, pp 217–254

Proudfoot W, Shaver P: Attribution theory and the psychology of religion. Journal for the Scientific Study of Religion 14:317–330, 1976

Sedman G, Hopkinson G: The psychopathology of mystical and religious conversion experiences in psychiatric patients, I, II. Confinia Psychiatrica (Basel) 9:1–19, 65–77, 1966

Singer M: Therapy with ex-cult members. National Association of Private Psychiatric Hospitals Journal 9(4):14–18, 1978

Sterba R: Remarks on mystic states. American Imago 25:77–85, 1968

Wenegrat B: Religious cult membership: a sociobiologic model, in Cults and New Religious Movements: A Report of the American Psychiatric Association. Edited by Galanter M. Washington, DC, American Psychiatric Association, 1989, pp 193–210

Wilson WP: Mental health benefits of religious salvation. Diseases of the Nervous System 33:383–386, 1972

SECTION II

❧

Treatment Issues at the Interface of Psychiatry and Religion

ເ໑ CHAPTER 5 ໑ວ

Psychiatric Therapies Influenced by Religious Movements

David R. Johnson, M.D., M.P.H., and
Joseph Westermeyer, M.D., M.P.H., Ph.D.

Treatment of the mentally ill began within the context of cultural "worldviews," tied largely to religious beliefs. The first healers were shamans who discharged many duties performed nowadays by clergy and physician-healers. Thus, religious, spiritual, and philosophical developments have influenced psychiatric therapies throughout history and, as we argue in this chapter, continue to do so today. In this chapter we describe these diverse influences on past and present psychiatric therapies. We specifically address those psychotherapies that have grown out of or been influenced by religious precepts, or that have evolved in tandem with specific religious movements—as contrasted with those therapies that have grown out of psychological theory (e.g., learning) or neuropsychiatric theory (e.g., neurotransmitters). Additionally, we discuss various psychotherapies with spiritual or philosophical roots, as well as mainstream psychiatric treatments that have incorporated religious concepts and structures. Finally, we explore

We acknowledge Jerome Kroll, M.D., for his review and suggestions.

specific treatment issues pertaining to psychotherapies that have been influenced by religious movements. As Kroll (1995) has pointed out, psychiatrists have often distanced themselves from, or even mistrusted, certain elements of religiosity. Thus, we believe it important that psychiatrists recognize the bases of religious thought in their own clinical work and the clinical work of others, so that they may consider the applicability of their concepts and clinical methods for their increasingly multicultural patient populations.

Religious Roots of Psychiatric Treatment

From earliest times to the present, healing has taken place in a sociocultural context. A central feature of this context in any society has been the religious belief and practice of the people (see Chapter 2 in this volume). Religion intimately affects a people's understanding of illness, healing, suffering, and death. Thus, healing and treatment in every culture throughout history have, at least in part, been founded in religion (see Chapter 1 in this volume). The following examples of prominent religious belief systems through the world are presented as a prelude to a discussion of therapeutics.

Prehistory and Early History

Throughout much of prehistory and even recent history, the shaman, priest, or native healer functioned as both religious and mental health specialist (Sevensky 1984). In many cultures, these personages still fill the dual role of psychological diagnostician and psychotherapeutic agent (Richardson 1978). This sociocultural convention has stemmed from the assumption that magical influences or malevolent deities cause mental illness. These beliefs about the preternatural causes of mental illness probably predated written history and were certainly present at the dawn of history in Egypt and the Near East. Priests were the main therapists, using religious and magical rites (incantations, herbal nostrums, physical therapies) to counter these supernatural forces. The Hebrews believed that madness was punishment by God for sin and that through their special relationship with God, priests had the ability to cure madness.

Animistic Religions

Animism continues to influence religious beliefs and practice throughout the world. Animists believe that anima, or spirits, exist throughout nature. Human beings are thought to possess one or more anima; loss of anima may be a cause of illness or even death. In addition, large trees, deep forests, imposing hills or mountains, rivers and lakes, and even large buildings or homes may each possess its own anima. Disrespect for or abuse of the physical environment may anger these anima-in-nature, provoking them to retaliate by causing illness, bad fortune, or death. Animals may have anima, which likewise sustain life but also cause mischief if disrespected or abused. Ghosts are simply the anima of people who have died; they may also inflict harm (Henderson and Adour 1981).

People may practice animism concurrently with one of the monotheistic religions (Tambiah 1975). Perhaps one of the better-known animistic religions of the world is Shinto in Japan. Much religious practice may be described as animistic or as some combination of animism and monotheism. Examples include many Native American religions, indigenous African religions, the religions of many Asian mountaineer peoples, and the practices of the ancient Greeks and Romans. In settings where both animistic shamanism and psychiatry are practiced, patients and their families may seek the assistance of both a shaman and a psychiatrist either concurrently or sequentially for a given problem. Although animism was once thought to be obsolete in the United States, immigration and internal migration have brought many thousands of animists to the offices of American psychiatrists (Gaviria and Wintrob 1979).

Several concepts are key to understanding the animistic patient in a psychiatric setting:

- The notion of anima existing not only within humans but also within animals and significant topographic features in the environment
- The ongoing reciprocal relationship between the living and the dead
- The special nature of sleep or "dream time" as comprising actual events in another world or another form of existence
- The idea of soul loss, the means by which soul loss can be induced, and the role of soul loss in the production of illness
- The means and mechanisms of curing spirit-induced illness

Buddhism

The premise that psychological misery is mainly symbolic or conceptual appeared early in the belief structure of Buddhism, one of the earliest of the world's "great religions" that is still practiced today by several hundred million people. Twenty-five hundred years ago in India, Gautama Buddha noted,

We are what we think. All that we are arises with our thoughts. With our thoughts, we make the world. Speak or act with an impure mind, and trouble will follow you, as the wheel follows the ox that draws the cart. (Byrom 1976, p. 3)

Buddha taught a simple system of the Four Noble Truths as the "middle way" toward Nirvana, or enlightenment. These concepts will be discussed in more detail later in this chapter when we consider the influence of various religious concepts on current schools of psychotherapy.

Ancient Greece

Plato (427–347 B.C.E.) conceived of the soul as composed of three parts: the rational, the spirited–affective, and the appetitive (Jowett 1937). This tripartite model has been compared to Freud's topographic concept of id, ego, and superego, as well as to Berne's parent-adult-child model (Berne 1961). Plato delineated two types of madness:

1. Madness from human ailments, in which the appetitive soul becomes dominant over the rational soul
2. Madness produced by divine disturbances of the soul, causing either inspired or destructive behavior

Plato prescribed music and a verbal dialectic between the patient and the physician. The goal of the dialectic was to alleviate the illness by enhancing knowledge—a concept analogous to Buddhist concepts evolving around the same time.

Other Greeks subsequently added to Plato's ideas. For example, Aristotle described the emotions as consisting of desire, anger, fear, courage, envy, joy, hatred, and pity (Ross 1955). Epicurean and Stoic philosophers believed that passions and unsatisfied desires acted on the soul to produce mental illnesses and that these illnesses could be controlled and avoided by attaining (via thoughts and conduct) a mental state of *ataraxia*, or lack of perturbation.

Influenced by earlier civilizations and surrounding peoples, the ancient Greeks evolved three psychological therapies for mental illnesses: therapy of words, induced sleep, and dream divination. Words used to promote healing could take multiple forms: prayers, magical incantations, cheering speeches, rhetorical speeches for persuasion, and Plato's verbal dialectics. Consolation, delivered through a speech, letter, or poem addressed to a grieving or depressed patient, was intended to help restore mental equilibrium. In-duced-sleep and dream-divination treatment involved different methods of suggestion. These treatments were provided by priests in sanctuaries and temples. Most notable of these sanctuaries was that of Asclepios, the god of healing. As members of the deity's cult, patients participated in temple activities, read votive tablets that reported other individuals' recoveries, and slept in an incubation room. In this incubation room, while dreaming or half-awake, they saw visions of Asclepios. The god might order certain remedies, command the dreamer to perform painful acts, or suggest that temple dogs or snakes lick the dreamer's body. Temple priests would interpret the dream and suggest further healing measures.

European and American Indian Influences in North America

During the early 19th century, many Americans, like their European counterparts, believed that mentally ill persons were possessed by the Devil. Diverse measures—prayer, cajoling, threats, physical punishment—were used to drive the devil out. The late-17th-century witch trials in Salem, Massachusetts, in which mentally ill persons constituted both victims and accusers, provide an extreme example of such beliefs, which persisted well into the 18th century. Little medical treatment and no organized services for mentally ill individuals existed during this period, and in the few instances in which mental illness was considered to be a medical problem, the underlying cause was regarded as excessive bile or disordered blood vessels. Venesections, purging, and blistering constituted the treatments of the time (Bell 1980; Deutsch 1949; Shryock 1944; Thompson 1994).

In general, the diverse American Indian groups throughout North America did not consider mental illness to be separate from physical illness and spiritual difficulties. Indian people focused on restoring health through rituals and prayers performed by medicine men and women rather than through attempts to expel demons from afflicted individuals. These ceremonies were the first "psychiatric" therapies performed on this continent by persons identified as healers. Although none of these pre–1500 C.E. modalities have yet entered the mainstream of psychiatric care, post–1500 C.E. modalities—composed of aboriginal Indian and European practices—have appeared, as detailed later in this chapter (Thompson et al. 1993; Walker and LaDue 1986).

The original peoples of the Americas used a method of life guidance broadly labeled as the Vision Quest. At particular junctures during life (and especially during young adulthood), individuals would seek life guidance during altered states of consciousness. Some groups employed fasting, sleep deprivation, and social isolation as a means of seeking such guidance, which might appear through auditory or visual hallucinations. Other groups used hallucinogenic substances, such as peyote, to help induce these experiences. The Native American Church evolved as an admixture of this ancient Vision Quest (using peyote to facilitate a personal "vision") and certain elements of Christianity (La Barre 1964; Opler 1942). These Christian elements included meeting at a particular time (often over a weekend) and place as a part of a group, conducting the ritual under the aegis of a leader, expressing one's personal experience in words to a group of fellow worshipers, and playing or listening to music (traditional native drumming and chanting). The spiritual ceremony was followed by a communal meal. Many Native Americans have found these religious practices useful in helping them deal with various life stressors, losses, and alcoholism (Albaugh and Anderson 1974; Bergman 1971; Hill 1990).

In the 1960s, on the basis of the Native American Church's experience with hallucinogens, lysergic acid diethylamide (LSD) and mescaline were examined for potential use in psychiatric treatment (Chandler and Harman 1960; Sherwood et al. 1962). Early studies of these agents were uncontrolled and involved a variety of patients (Savage et al. 1966). These studies generated considerable optimism for LSD in the treatment of alcoholism (Kurland et al. 1967). Consequently, the use of LSD in the treatment of alcoholic individuals was scientifically studied (Ludwig et al. 1969). However, careful analysis of LSD in a research format failed to show any efficacy. In addition, many patients had transient psychosis and/or "flashbacks" after LSD. One could argue that these studies were flawed, given that LSD is a potent synthetic hallucinogen and administration occurred in a clinical setting (whereas folk use involved naturally occurring, weaker hallucinogens administered in a religious setting). Nonetheless, the results of these LSD studies have not encouraged others to repeat such trials.

The Influence of Religious Beliefs on Psychiatric Care

Psychotherapy With Animistic Patients

The notion of soul loss or soul injury as a cause of illness requires that the patient (and the clinician) deal with illness as a spiritual or religious phenomenon. The clinician may also need to address spiritual or ethical concerns as part of treatment. Moral and existential questions may arise during the process of understanding the illness, as well as in subsequent treatment (Westermeyer 1988).

This combined psychospiritual approach can provide potential therapeutic benefits by fostering holistic thinking, hopefulness, and acceptance in the patient and family. Animists may accept unsuccessful treatment and even death without the sense of failure that is apt to overwhelm rationalistic (as opposed to rational) or scientistic (as opposed to scientific) patients and clinicians. Nonanimists may refer to this phenomenon as "fatalism," but it is less a negative indifference than a measured acceptance (Westermeyer 1989).

Injury to or loss of one's anima implies that the individual's vital life force has been diminished in an essential fashion. By extrapolation, rehabilitation or recovery involves a deep-seated "resurrection" of the individual's spiritual and vital forces, not just a healing of tissues and a normalization of physiological processes. As a consequence, animistic patients and families are often prepared, by dint of their basic notions about life and living, to undertake the fundamental changes that recovery from major mental illness often requires.

Clinicians may employ animistic viewpoints to enhance their patients' understanding in various types of psychotherapy. For the therapist undertaking insight-oriented therapy, an understanding of both the patient's clinical condition and the patient's worldview is critical. Because this type of therapy involves analogies taken from the patient's life experience and culture, the clinician must appreciate the patient's cultural symbols and their meanings. In behavioral modification–based and rational–emotive therapies, on the other hand, knowledge of the patient's worldview is not as crucial, although an understanding of the patient's clinical condition is still important. These modalities are not so reliant on cultural norms, values, myths, and understandings.

For the therapist familiar with the animistic patient's view of the world, the use of culturally appropriate therapeutic interventions is virtually unavoidable. The therapist is not so much applying unique therapeutic interventions as applying well-known, familiar therapeutic interventions that are culturally consistent with the patient's worldview. Unlike shamanistic healing practices, which tend to involve absolute prescriptions and assertions of fact, these psychotherapeutic interventions make use of the patient's worldview to discover alternative formulations conducive to recovery. The therapist's interpretations are geared toward enhancing patients' self-understanding and providing them with control over their destinies. Rather than assuming a shamanistic stance, in which the patient is directed by the healer, the clinician assists the patient in becoming *self*-directed. The goal is an independent patient who can use animistic concepts to deal with changing personal and environmental circumstances. To help the patient achieve this goal, the clinician must appreciate the nature of animistic thinking, along with its advantages and potential pitfalls for the psychiatric patient.

Moral Treatment

Animistic theories about mental illness imply a need to take action against the presumed pathogenic anima. Interventions could be supportive and caring if the therapist were attempting to strengthen a beneficent but weakened anima. On the other hand, therapeutic efforts could be damaging or detrimental to the patient if they were directed at forcing out an "evil" or pathogenic anima or destroying a demonic anima that presumably had taken possession of the patient. Consequently, animistic therapists might treat mentally ill persons in harsh ways (e.g., imprisonment, restraint, punishment, torture, burning). With the appearance of moral treatment, the therapist—regardless of his or her theories about etiology—committed to a benign, considerate, even respectful approach to mentally ill people.

During the 16th and 17th centuries, a growing secular interest in the natural world displaced the European religions of the day from their hegemony over philosophy, epistemology, and science. One might argue that religious emphasis on moral behavior, and even later on social morality, occurred in this context of waning church influence over knowledge and scientific progress. The religious emphasis on morality, in turn, influenced secular society through its influence on cultural mores and social movements. By the late 17th and early 18th centuries, these moral changes in secular society were having effects on the treatment of the mentally ill.

Moral treatment began in Europe and North America in post-Renaissance Catholic/Christian settings. The moral treatment movements in these regions occurred at a time when humanistic values upholding the dignity of each individual were emerging. It is perhaps no coincidence that the earliest attempts to establish democratic or republican governments free of inherited kingships were also beginning. Cartesian notions of the mind as separate from the body (i.e., mind–body dualism) were also just appearing. Thus, moral treatment can be seen as reflecting an admixture of religious belief and principle, secular values emphasizing the individual apart from the collective, and political movements in which individual achievement was valued over socially ascribed status.

It was in this historical context that the French physician Philippe Pinel (1745–1826) initiated dramatic and much-publicized changes in the asylum treatment of mental illness (Pinel 1801/1962). He removed the chains from the insane (as persons with mental illness were designated) and began an asylum regimen in which patients were treated kindly (although threats and other pressures were sometimes used). Efforts were made to meet the special needs of patients through occupational therapy, exercise, entertainment, good food, and attractive surroundings. He also instituted regular meetings of hospital attendants with groups of patients. Pinel called his approach to care the moral treatment of insanity, and he believed it would be curative. Moral treatment represented the application of the French concepts of enlightenment through education, reason, and persuasion. Furthermore, it was built on Pinel's rejection of humoral, spiritual, and animistic theories of mental illness etiology. Parenthetically, Pinel's *Treatise on Insanity* (published in 1801) contained excellent descriptions of the major symptoms of insanity for his time. In the book he recognized four forms of mental illness—mania, melancholia, dementia, and idiocy—and described the natural history and response to treatment of each.

During the 1790s, the Englishman William Tuke (1732–1819), influenced by the ideas of Pinel, founded the York Retreat (Tuke 1813/1964). Somewhat later, Benjamin Rush (1745–1813) petitioned for humanitarian reforms in the treatment of the mentally ill at Pennsylvania Hospital, the first United States hospital to admit psychiatric patients. Rush improved the hospital setting by adding heating and ventilation to wards; separating out violent patients; adding work, exercise, and amusement activities to patients' daily routines; excluding visitors who might disturb patients; and hiring better-trained staff. Although he believed that mentally ill individuals should be freed from moral stigma and housed decently, Rush relied on some traditional coercive treatments: physical restraint, chastisement, and whirling in a rotary chair (Rush 1812).

The first American asylum exclusively for mentally ill patients opened in Williamsburg, Virginia in the late 1770s. In 1817, a second asylum, Friends Hospital, was established north of Philadelphia by the Quakers. Founded on the principles of moral treatment set forth by William Tuke in England, this hospital used no chains or other extreme forms of restraint, and violent patients were placed on a separate floor.

Moral treatment was practiced by the superintendents of asylums because of a faith, inspired by Pinel and by the York Retreat, that it could cure many early cases of insanity. The asylum movement and moral treatment were further stimulated by the endeavors of lay reformers, most notably Dorothea Dix (1802–1887), who devoted her life to exposing the maltreatment of patents in psychiatric institutions (Caplan 1969; Deutsch 1949; Walker and LaDue 1986).

The era of moral treatment has continued to this day. However, several events of the last few decades suggest that North America (and other societies) may be moving away from the movement's original guiding principles. Among mentally ill persons, homelessness, relegation to harsh survival on the streets, and denial of needed psychiatric treatment have resulted from an apparent shift in societal values away from the principles inherent in moral treatment. It is perhaps no coincidence that, in the midst of growing societal indifference to suffering, self-help movements have evolved and flourished. Paradoxically, some psychiatrists have begun to identify with specific religious beliefs or practices.

Christian Psychiatry and Religious Healing

Modern Christian healing movements appeal to the New Testament's authority, citing examples of healing contained in the Gospels (Favazza 1982). Healing, and especially healing of mental illness caused by demonic possession, was a large aspect of Jesus' ministry. Over the centuries, however, Christianity's healing function was superseded by the notion that spiritual salvation was primary and bodily suffering was noble. Despite general neglect of the Christian healing tradition, certain holy healing shrines were established. For example, the Shrine of St. Dymphna in Gheel, Belgium, was associated with the healing of mental illness.

The modern Pentecostal religious movement began in 1900 after Charles F. Parham, a Methodist minister, brought together a group of friends in an attempt to discover the secret of early Christians (Sherill 1977). This group re-initiated attempts to heal illness through spiritual means. Initially, the Pentecostal and other Fundamentalist Protestants engaging in faith healing were primarily rural and blue collar. More recently, however, the practice of faith healing has become middle class. In 1978, 2,500 Catholic and Episcopal churches reportedly had regular spiritual healing services. Alcoholism, gambling, and emotional disorders have been labeled as today's demons. In *The Christian's Handbook of Psychiatry*, a psychiatrist has written that demonic possession is primarily a spiritual problem, with physical and psychotic manifestations as incidental by-products (Hyden 1973).

Christian faith healers often use a simplified form of psychodynamic psychotherapy, prayers, and the use of a lifelong support system through participation in a Christian community. These Christian groups are similar in many ways to mutual-help associations found in many cultures: Alcoholics Anonymous, Zar cults in Eastern Africa, and Puerto Rican Spiritualist Centros. Most influential modern faith healers encourage people to seek medical and/or psychiatric help. "Christian" psychiatrists are usually the preferred resource.

Gaines (1982), who studied self-avowed Christian psychiatrists, concluded that there is no unified "Christian Psychiatry." He noted that the "Christian" aspect of the typical Christian psychiatrist pertains to a personal religious experience—that is, a "second birth" from which has developed an ongoing, personal relationship with Christ. In his study of Christian psychiatrists at a Southern teaching hospital, Gaines found a significant diversity of beliefs about prayer and healing. All Christian psychiatrists at this center prayed for at least some of their patients; however, not all prayed with their patients. Those who did pray with patients noted that they would not initiate prayer without clear signs from the patient as to its appropriateness. These psychiatrists also noted certain circumstances in which they might deny a request for prayer from a patient in therapy.

Debate about value neutrality in psychotherapy has arisen from consideration of Christian psychiatrists as well as those performing any type of psychotherapy (Sevensky 1984). The notion that a moral life is important to mental health has spread beyond the original group of Christian psychiatrists. Popular radio talk-show psychologist Dr. Laura Schlessinger, who draws more than 10 million listeners weekly, has remarked that her show is not a mental health show but a "moral health show" (Bernstein 1996). In rejecting the notion that feelings are paramount, she observed: "in the last 20 or 30 years, we erected a monument to feelings and made them the vantage point from which to make decisions. That's dangerous."

Indeed, the religious beliefs of therapists are generally liberal relative to those of the population as a whole (Henry et al. 1971). In a random sample of American Psychological Association psychologists, 50% reported that they believed in God, in contrast to 90% of the general population. Of interest in this regard, Azhar and colleagues (1994) observed that patients with anxiety disorder showed significantly more rapid improvement in symptoms with "religious psychotherapy" than with supportive psychotherapy and medication. Propst and co-workers (1992) similarly found that depressed patients receiving religious-content cognitive-behavioral therapy (RCT) and pastoral counseling therapy (PCT) reported significantly lower posttreatment depression and adjustment scores (correlating with improvement in depressive symptoms and functioning) than did either the nonreligious cognitive-behavioral therapy (NRCT) or the waiting-list control (WLC) group. However, after 3 months, and at 2-year follow up, the RCT, PCT, and NRCT groups showed equal improvement—which was greater than the improvement in the posttreatment WLC group.

Of relevance to this topic is the work of Mollica et al. (1986), who noted that clergy referred less than 10% of their counselees to specialized mental health resources. Taggart (1973) has described a change in pastoral counseling since 1960. This change has included a shift away from parish-based counseling to counseling centers or medical settings, a declining interest in traditional religious practices and convictions, an increased interest in psychological practices and theories, the charging of fees, and increased institutional barriers to individuals who are perceived as inappropriate for counseling or who are unable to pay.

Self-Help Movements

During the last century, as social and medical institutions have proven ineffective or uninterested in addressing certain human ills, various self-help movements have evolved. These movements clearly have their roots in the Christian religion, although other religious faiths have adopted their concepts and methods. These 20th-century movements may be traced to ancient and modern religion-based charitable orders, such as the Knights of Malta, the Knights of Columbus, the Red Cross (among Christians), and the Red Crescent (among Muslims). However, these latter-day self-help groups have had as their goal the betterment of the self (as victim of alcoholism or other malady) rather than the betterment of others-as-victims (e.g., of war, catastrophe, slavery).

Alcoholics Anonymous.   Founded in 1935, Alcoholics Anonymous (AA) had its origin in the transcendent religious experience of its principal founder, Bill W. (Glaser 1974). Bill W., an individual suffering from severe alcohol dependence, was visited by a friend who belonged to the Oxford Group. Originally known as the First Century Christian Fellowship, the Oxford Group was founded by Dr. Frank Nathan Daniel Buchman around 1921. Dr. Buchman, a Lutheran clergyman in Pennsylvania, experienced a mystical enlightenment regarding original Christianity before the organized church (hence the name First Century Christian Fellowship). Practices of the Oxford Group Movement included "sharing," "guidance," "changing," and "making restitution" (Barry 1932; Campbell 1972):

- *Sharing* meant the open confession of sins, frequently at large meetings. *Sin* meant an improper action rather than a doctrinal deviation in thought or speech.
- *Guidance* meant the acceptance of divine inspiration as the sole indication of what one should do.

- *Changing*, or conversion to the beliefs of the Oxford Group, was considered essential. Conversion was described as a sudden, dramatic, emotional, and often public experience—not unlike a revelation. Once a person had been "changed," he or she would be free from sin for the rest of his life, or "second born."
- *Making restitution* meant that repentance of sins was not enough; one must do something to make amends for past actions.

The Oxford Group movement also attempted to instill "absolute values"—that is, absolute honesty, purity, unselfishness, and love—in its members.

Under the guidance of the Oxford Group, Bill W. achieved sobriety. He joined the New York Calgary Church Parish House branch led by Dr. Samuel Shoemaker (an Episcopal clergyman), about whom Bill W. subsequently wrote:

> . . . the early AA got its ideas of self-examination, acknowledgment of character defects, restitution for harm done, and working with others straight from the Oxford Groups and directly from Sam Shoemaker, their former leader in America, and from nowhere else. (W. 1957, p. 39)

AA meetings, similar to the Oxford Group, employed ritualized open confessions of prior transgressions and the acceptance of a "Higher Power" for guidance. Ten of the Twelve Steps of Alcoholics Anonymous are based on the Oxford Group creed. Openly acknowledging one's helplessness before alcohol and carrying the message to other alcoholic individuals are unique to AA.

Synanon. The first of the drug-free therapeutic communities, Synanon was founded in California (1958) by Charles E. Dederich III, an AA member (Yablonsky 1965). Dederich attempted to adopt AA's techniques for narcotic addicts. However, he made profound and original innovations himself. He introduced "attack therapy," or encounter-type groups. Synanon was the first self-help movement to be exclusively residential in nature. In place of a God-centered theology, Synanon espoused a kind of "secular theology" (i.e., a change from Religion to religion and from theology to sociology). The Synanon experience began with inductees severing all ties with outsiders for 3 months, after which they lived in isolated settings. There, they worked in Synanon-operated businesses—specifically to remove them from community influences that might rekindle heroin cravings. Members usually spent about 30 hours each month in group encounters called "games." During these meetings, harsh dialogue and confrontation were employed to convert the addict to a new style of living, to act as a safety valve for communal animosities, and to ensure members' compliance with group demands. Synanon later suffered as a result of the concentration of organizational power in Dederich's hands. Later, New York's Daytop Village (1964), its offshoot Gaudenzia Incorporated of Philadelphia (1968), and other groups developed along the lines of Synanon.

Morita Therapy

Morita therapy bears some resemblance to North American inpatient psychiatric practices of the late 1970s, when mean lengths of stay ranged from several weeks to a few months and hospitalization was oriented toward providing respite and asylum. Since then, inpatient psychiatric treatment has adopted a much more rapid, even frenetic pace. Patients are expected to face their problems, consider their alternatives, and leave the hospital with a therapeutic plan within several days. Nonetheless, certain principles of Morita therapy can be applied to day programs and outpatient clinics (see section below titled "Buddhism and Cognitive-Behavioral Therapy for Borderline Personality Disorder").

Elements of Morita therapy can be traced to the religions, philosophies, and "worldviews" that have held sway for centuries in Japan. The ancient animistic Shinto religion, still actively practiced in Japan today, preaches a respect for, melding with, and peaceful connection to the natural world. Confucian features are evident in the powerful role of the therapist, who isolates the patient from human society, provides shelter and nourishment, and then both teaches and guides the patient back to wholeness. Taoist concepts appear in the emphasis on process and acceptance, and in the central role accorded to social forces in recovering one's mental health. Zen Buddhism prescribes acceptance, simplicity, and humility—together with respect for self and others—on the road back to wellness. These belief systems, all still powerful in Japan and often practiced concurrently by the same individual, serve as conceptual foundations for Morita therapy.

In 1917, Professor Shomei Morita of Jikei University in Japan published a paper describing a method of treatment now referred to as Morita therapy. The practice of Morita therapy in Japan bears a striking resemblance to the practices of drug-free therapeutic communities in the United States. Interestingly, both therapeutic systems were derived from religious sources: Professor Morita's methods developed from Zen Buddhism, and the methods of therapeutic communities evolved from charismatic/evangelical Protestantism (Kora 1965; Kora and Ohara 1973). The Morita method also resembles certain features of Western obstetrical treatment for hyperemesis gravidarum (i.e., hospitalization in a quiet, darkened room without visitors; respite from responsibilities and labors; social isolation; reduced external stimuli; therapeutic control of diet and physical exertion; instruction on diet and behavior; gradual resumption of social and occupational activities).

Morita therapy, although it has been of some help to patients with mild psychotic disorders and drug addiction, has proven most applicable to personality neuroses called *shinkeishitsu*. There are three types of *shinkeishitsu* (Kora 1965):

1. Neurasthenia, which includes insomnia, hypochondriasis and multiple somatic complaints;
2. Anxiety neurosis, which includes anxiety, fear, and some panic disorder symptoms; and
3. Obsessional fears, mainly of imperfection or embarrassment (Kora 1965).

All three maladies receive similar treatment.

The *shinkeishitsushu* illness develops in those who are introverted, nervous, overanxious, and shy. It represents a character-related response to a particular encounter with the environment. For example, a man who experienced dizziness following an extended soak at a Japanese public bath developed an intense fear of reexperiencing the dizziness and could not return to public bathing. This then prevented his adjustment to his life by interfering with his ability to cope with a common demand (i.e., that he attend public baths with his relatives and friends).

The morbid fear of blushing is usually the core or overwhelming *shinkeishitsushu* symptom. The typical person with *shinkeishitsushu* is shy and timid, but often extremely ambitious as well. Such people cannot accept the passive solution to their problem by simply retreating from an active social life. They usually have extraordinarily strong drives to be better than others, to contribute to the world's knowledge, to be rich, to hold high social position, and so forth. These individuals also tend to be intellectually oriented and academically high achievers. Such patients tend to use their intellectual gifts to analyze their apparent imperfections and to criticize themselves unmercifully. Attention is focused on some symptom (e.g., dizziness or blushing), and thus the symptom is exacerbated. Morita therapy deconditions the symptoms by concentrating on them (Kora and Ohara 1973), a paradoxical intervention within a context supported by traditional beliefs, values, and roles.

In Morita therapy, the therapist assists patients in gaining "insight" into the nature or essence of all things (Kora 1965). The patient is encouraged to identify with nature and to see how foolish it is to struggle against hate or fear. To have insight into true nature is to achieve an attitude of living in harmony with the universe. Morita summarized his concept in the Japanese word *arugamama* (meaning "as it is"). *Arugamama* is a form of enlightenment, or *satori* in Zen Buddhism. In Morita therapy, as individuals achieve their personal *satori* (e.g., "I am a coward"), they no longer need to pretend that they are brave, and can live as they are. The rationale consists of attaining *arugamama*, just as practiced in Zen, releasing behavior from the interference of the resistive, doubting, observational self. The release is through self-acceptance at a less-than-perfect level—that is, one becomes satisfied with what one can do rather than being obsessed with what one must do. Release involves freedom from an internalized family superego that demands more than an individual can deliver (Kora 1965).

Buddhism and Psychotherapy

Buddhism has had profound and diverse effects on various psychiatric therapies for over 2,000 years. Buddhism is at once a religion, a philosophical system, and an ancient psychology of thought and action. The originator of Buddhist thought, Siddhartha Gautama, taught a simple system of the "Four Noble Truths" (MacHovec 1984):

- Existence is painful; to live is to know pain; no one is spared pain.
- The reason for and source of pain lie within one's self.
- Suffering and pain need not be so; not for you, for others, or for the world.
- The way to transcendence lies between excess and deprivation.

Buddha taught an Eightfold Path containing behavioral and humanistic concepts. These concepts focus on the nature of perception, cognitive restructuring, attitudes and assumptions, coping skills, goal setting, and value clarification. Elements of the Eightfold Path (described further in Chapter 1 of this volume) are Right View, Right Resolve, Right Speech (and Silence), Right Conduct, Right Livelihood, Right Effort, Right Awareness, and Right Meditation.

Buddhist practices have many similarities with various psychiatric therapies practiced in North America. For example, Fritz Perls referred to "the immediacy of experiencing" as "mini-satoris" (*satori* translates roughly to "enlightenment") and conceded that he gained as much insight from his study of Zen Buddhism as from his years with Freud (Smith 1976). Erich

Fromm and his colleagues wrote a book on Zen Buddhism and contemporary psychoanalysis (Suzuki et al. 1963). Werner Erhard, the leader of the popular self-help movement Est (Erhard Seminar Training), has publicly acknowledged the movement's conceptual indebtedness to Buddhism (Bartley 1978). Cognitive-behavioral therapy techniques such as relaxation training and imagery work also have strong similarities to Buddhist techniques (Watts 1961). Linehan (1993a, 1993b) has used certain Buddhist techniques in her cognitive-behavioral therapy for borderline personality disorder (see below).

Buddhism and Cognitive-Behavioral Therapy for Borderline Personality Disorder

Marsha Linehan has developed a therapy she describes as an integration of two areas: her work in suicide prevention and behavior therapy and her experience as a Zen student of a Zen master and Benedictine monk (Linehan 1993a, 1993b). The main goals of Linehan's therapy are to enhance dialectical patterns of cognitive functioning and to change extreme behaviors to more balanced and integrated responses to the moment. Dialectical Behavior Therapy (DBT) does not focus on maintaining a stable, consistent environment, but instead aims to help the patient become comfortable with change. According to Linehan, the three main polarities of DBT are 1) the need for patients to accept themselves as they are and the need to change; 2) the tension between patients' getting what they need and losing what they need if they become more competent; and 3) patients' maintaining personal integrity versus learning new skills that will help them emerge from their suffering.

Linehan has described dialectical thinking as the "middle path" between universalistic thinking and relativistic thinking. Dialectical thinking assumes that truth and order evolve and develop over time. Goals of this process consist of integrating contradictory points of view, learning to be comfortable with inconsistency, and avoiding simplistic explanations. This method is applied to patients with borderline personality disorder, who often have difficulty receiving new information and who tend to search unsuccessfully for absolute truths. Extremes and rigid behavior patterns are signals that a "middle way" has not been achieved.

Linehan explains that the paradox of change versus acceptance runs throughout her therapy; all behavior is "good," yet the patient is in therapy to change "bad" behavior. Through paradox, therapists highlight the seeming incongruity that even the inability to accept must be accepted. DBT teaches four crisis-survival strategies: self-soothing, distracting, improving the moment, and thinking of pros and cons.

Eastern Contemplative Traditions and Transpersonal Psychotherapy

Hindu and Buddhist psychologies primarily address existential and transpersonal levels of being; they lack any detailed analyses of areas such as early development, psychodynamics, and the unconscious. They also appear to have relatively little to offer those with severe psychological disturbances. In contrast, Hindu and Buddhist psychologies contain detailed maps of states of consciousness, peak experiences, and developmental levels, although these phenomena seemingly lie beyond traditional Western psychological descriptions (Burtt 1955).

The transpersonal movement began in the San Francisco Bay area in the late 1960s, when a small group of people began to meet with the goal of expanding the scope of Western psychology (Hutton 1994; Walsh 1988, 1993). They believed that Western psychology and culture were overlooking some of the most important and meaningful dimensions of human existence. Psychological health or exceptional well-being had received little attention from psychologists and psychiatrists. Dimensions of human experience such as spirituality and altered states of consciousness had been reduced or pathologized to neurotic immaturities or random neuronal firings. Mystical experience and enlightenment were often dismissed as regression to intrauterine stages. In response to these views, Wilber (1977, 1980) has argued that major differences exist between pathological ego dissolution (pre-egoic regression) and trans-egoic disidentification (trans-subject/object states). In the latter, the individual can transcend subject and object while remaining aware of conventional reality.

Abraham Maslow (1968) also played a central role in the genesis of the transpersonal movement with his interest in psychological health. His finding that "self-actualizers," or exceptionally healthy subjects, tended to have "peak experiences" (spontaneous, ecstatic, unitive states of consciousness akin to "mystic experiences") catalyzed the birth of the transpersonal movement (Walsh 1993). Early on, it was thought that peak experiences were inevitably spontaneous, brief, and virtually overwhelming. However, early transpersonal movement pioneers were amazed to find detailed accounts not just of peak experiences, but of whole families of peak experiences and systematic techniques to induce and sustain these. This information was mainly found in Asian psychologies, philosophies, religions, and contemplative disciplines. Transpersonal psychologists have also attempted to experimentally examine advanced stages of Buddhist meditation as well as lucid dreaming (Brown et al. 1984; Shapiro and Walsh 1984).

Conclusions

Religion is inseparable from societal views of proper behavior, psychological well-being, and the meaning of suffering. Self-help groups employ these principles, as do many caregivers with whom psychiatrists have cause to interact (e.g., clergy, therapists from other disciplines, so-called folk healers). Moreover, many psychiatric therapies employ values, concepts, and even therapeutic methods that have originated from religious beliefs and practices. The skilled psychiatrist practicing in a multiethnic, multireligious society appreciates the religious influences that have shaped modern psychiatric practice. Potential strengths and weaknesses exist in the religious and philosophical beliefs that our patients bring to the clinical setting—or that they adopt in an effort to achieve some level of comfort or to provide meaning for their suffering. The worldviews undergirding our modern therapies rely on society's ability to accept and even support them. Patients or therapists sometimes denigrate worthwhile therapeutic approaches derived from religious or philosophical traditions different from their own.

Even with the evolution and progression of the scientific method, it is unlikely that genetics and neuroscience will ever be capable of fully explaining disturbances in thought, action, and intention of the human mind. Our minds are inextricably interwoven with and influenced by the social and cultural forces around us. Existential, spiritual, and religious concerns account for a large portion of these sociocultural forces. Understanding the individual's worldview will remain essential to the comprehensive study of human behavior and psychopathology.

References

Albaugh B, Anderson P: Peyote in the treatment of alcoholism among American Indians. Am J Psychiatry 131:1247–1256, 1974

Azhar MZ, Varma SL, Dharap AS: Religious psychotherapy in anxiety disorder patients. Acta Psychiatr Scand 90:1–3, 1994

Barry FR: The Oxford Group movement. The Spectator 149:147–148, 1932

Bartley W: Werner Erhard: The Founding of Est. New York, CN Potter, 1978

Bell LV: Treating the Mentally Ill From Colonial Times to the Present. New York, Praeger, 1980

Bergman RL: Navaho peyote use: its apparent safety. Am J Psychiatry 128:695–699, 1971

Berne E: Transactional Analysis in Psychotherapy. New York, Grove Press, 1961

Bernstein A: Dr. Laura's "Moral Health Show." U.S. News and World Report, April 29, 1996, p 22

Brown D, Forte M, Dysart M: Differences in visual sensitivity among mindfulness meditators and non-meditators. Percept Mot Skills 58:727–733, 1984

Burtt EA: The Teachings of the Compassionate Buddha. New York, Mentor Books, 1955

Byrom T: The Dhammapada. New York, Alfred A Knopf, 1976

Campbell J: Myths to Live By. New York, Viking, 1972

Caplan RB: Psychiatry and the Community in Nineteenth-Century America: The Recurring Concern With the Environment in the Prevention and Treatment of Mental Illness. New York, Basic Books, 1969

Chandler AL, Harman MA: LSD as a facilitating agent in psychotherapy. Arch Gen Psychiatry 2:286–300, 1960

Deutsch A: The Mentally Ill in America: A History of Their Care and Treatment from Colonial Times. New York, Columbia University Press, 1949

Favazza AR: Modern Christian healing of mental illness. Am J Psychiatry 139:728–735, 1982

Gaines AD: The twice-born: "Christian psychiatry" and Christian psychiatrists. Cult Med Psychiatry 6:305–324, 1982

Gaviria M, Wintrob RM: Spiritist or psychiatrist: treatment of mental illness among Puerto Ricans in two Connecticut towns. J Operational Psychiatry 10:40–46, 1979

Glaser FB: Some historical aspects of the drug-free therapeutic community. Am J Drug Alcohol Abuse 1:37–52, 1974

Henderson JN, Adour KK: Comanche ghost sickness: a biocultural perspective. Med Anthropol 5:195–205, 1981

Henry WE, Sims JH, Spray SL: The Fifth Profession: Becoming a Psychotherapist. San Francisco, CA, Jossey-Bass, 1971

Hill TW: Peyotism and the control of heavy drinking: the Nebraska Winnebago in the early 1900s. Human Organization 49(3):255–265, 1990

Hutton MS: How transpersonal psychotherapists differ from other practitioners: an empirical study. Journal of Transpersonal Psychology 26:139–148, 1994

Hyden OQ: The Christian's Handbook of Psychiatry. Old Tappan, NJ, Spire Books, 1973

Jowett B (tr): The Dialogues of Plato. New York, Random House, 1937

Kora T: Morita therapy. International Journal of Psychiatry 1:611–645, 1965

Kora T, Ohara K: Morita therapy. Psychology Today 6(16):63–68, 1973

Kroll J: Religion and psychiatry. Curr Opin Psychiatry 8:335–339, 1995

Kurland AA, Unger S, Shaffer JW: Psychedelic therapy utilizing LSD in the treatment of the alcoholic patient: a preliminary report. Am J Psychiatry 123:1202–1209, 1967

La Barre W: The Peyote Cult. Hamden, CT, Shoestring Press, 1964

Linehan MM: Cognitive-Behavioral Treatment of Borderline Personality Disorder. New York, Guilford, 1993a

Linehan MM: Skills Training Manual for Treating Borderline Personality Disorder. New York, Guilford, 1993b

Ludwig A, Levine J, Stark L, et al: A clinical study of LSD treatment in alcoholism. Am J Psychiatry 126:59–69, 1969

MacHovec FJ: Current therapies and the Ancient East. Am J Psychother 38:87–96, 1984

Maslow A: Toward a Psychology of Being. Princeton, NJ, Van Nostrand, 1968

Mollica RF, Streets FJ, Boscarino J, et al: A community study of formal pastoral counseling activities of the clergy. Am J Psychiatry 143:323–328, 1986

Opler M: Fact and fancy in Ute peyotism. American Anthropologist 44:151–159, 1942

Pinel P: A Treatise on Insanity (in Which Are Contained the Principles of a New and More Practical Nosology of Mental Disorders) (1801). Translated by Davis DD. New York, Hafner, 1962

Propst LR, Ostrom R, Watkins P, et al: Comparative efficacy of religious and nonreligious cognitive-behavioral therapy for the treatment of clinical depression in religious individuals. J Consult Clin Psychol 60:94–103, 1992

Richardson WJ: Religion and mental health, in The Encyclopedia of Bioethics. Edited by Reich WT. New York, Free Press, 1978, pp 1064–1070

Ross WD: Aristotle. London, Methuen, 1955

Rush B: Medical Inquiries and Observations Upon the Diseases of the Mind. Philadelphia, PA, Kimber & Richardson, 1812

Savage C, Fadiman J, Mogar R, et al: The effects of psychedelic (LSD) therapy on values, personality, and behavior. International Journal of Neuropsychiatry 2:241–254, 1966

Sevensky RL: Religion, psychology, and mental health. Am J Psychother 38:73–86, 1984

Shapiro D, Walsh R (eds): Meditation: Classic and Contemporary Perspectives. New York, Aldine, 1984

Sherill JL: They Speak With Other Tongues. Old Tappan, NJ, Revell (Spire Books), 1977

Sherwood JN, Stolaroff MJ, Harman WW: The psychedelic experience—a new concept in psychotherapy. J Neuropsychiatry 4:96–107, 1962

Shryock RH: The beginnings: from colonial days to the foundation of the American Psychiatric Association, in One Hundred Years of American Psychiatry. Edited by Hall JK, Zilboorg G, Burker HA. New York, Columbia University Press, 1944, pp 1–28

Smith EW (ed): The Growing Edge of Gestalt Therapy. New York, Brunner/Mazel, 1976

Suzuki D, Fromm E, DeMartino R (eds): Zen Buddhism and Psychoanalysis. New York, Grove, 1963

Taggart M: The professionalization of the parish pastoral counselor. Journal of Pastoral Care 27:180–188, 1973

Tambiah SJ: Buddhism and the Spirit Cults of North-East Thailand. Cambridge, UK, Cambridge University Press, 1975

Thompson JW: Trends in the development of psychiatric services; 1844–1994. Hospital and Community Psychiatry 45:987–992, 1994

Thompson JW, Walker RD, Silk-Walker P: Mental illness in American Indians and Alaska Natives, in Culture, Ethnicity, and Mental Illness. Edited by Gaw AC. Washington, DC, American Psychiatric Press, 1993, pp 189–243

Tuke S: Description of the Retreat (1813). London, Dawsons of Pall Mall, 1964

W. Bill: Alcoholics Anonymous Comes of Age: A Brief History of A.A. New York, Alcoholics Anonymous World Services, 1957

Walker RD, LaDue R: An integrative approach to American Indian mental health, in Ethnic Psychiatry. Edited by Wilkinson CB. New York, Plenum, 1986

Walsh R: Two Asian psychologies and their implications for Western psychotherapists. Am J Psychother 42:543–560, 1988

Walsh R: The transpersonal movement: a history and state of the art. Journal of Transpersonal Psychology 25:123–139, 1993

Watts A: Psychotherapy East and West. New York, Ballantine, 1961

Westermeyer J: Folk medicine in Laos: a comparison of two ethnic groups. Soc Sci Med 27:769–778, 1988

Westermeyer J: The Psychiatric Care of Migrants: A Clinical Guide. Washington, DC, American Psychiatric Press, 1989

Wilber K: The Spectrum of Consciousness. Wheaton, IL, Quest, 1977

Wilber K: The Atman Project: A Transpersonal View of Human Development. Wheaton, IL, Quest, 1980

Yablonsky L: The Tunnel Back: Synanon. New York, Macmillan, 1965

⁊⊙ CHAPTER 6 ⊙⁊

Moral and Spiritual Issues Following Traumatization

Landy F. Sparr, M.D., M.A., and
John F. Fergueson, M.Div.

In the past several decades, there has been considerable scientific interest in the psychological impact of severe stressors. With the advent of the third edition of the American Psychiatric Association's *Diagnostic and Statistical Manual of Mental Disorders* (DSM-III) in 1980, a new diagnostic category, posttraumatic stress disorder (PTSD), pulled together a previously diverse and heterogeneous nomenclature dating back more than 100 years. Since then, despite moderate debate about the diagnostic criteria for the condition and some slight modifications in subsequent DSM editions (DSM-III-R [American Psychiatric Association 1987] and DSM-IV [American Psychiatric Association 1994]), the validity of the core elements of the disorder has received plentiful empirical support (Sparr 1995).

The burgeoning literature on PTSD includes a body of research illustrating not only the wide range of the disorder's psychological effects but also the

---

The views and recommendations expressed in this chapter are those of the author and do not necessarily reflect official Department of Veterans Affairs policy.

The author wishes to thank Ms. Jackie Lockwood for her valuable assistance in manuscript preparation.

possibility that psychologically traumatic events induce lasting biological changes in exposed individuals. As Horowitz (1993) first systematically elucidated, the signs and symptoms of response to a severely traumatic life event are expressed in two predominant phases: 1) intrusive states, characterized by unbidden ideas, feelings, and even compulsive actions; and 2) denial states, characterized by emotional numbing and constriction of ideation. This biphasic response pattern is by now familiar to researchers and clinicians alike and has been incorporated into the diagnostic criteria. Not included in the DSM criteria but frequently cited in the trauma literature is a recognition of the major role religion and spirituality play in both development of and recovery from PTSD (Carmil and Breznitz 1991; Decker 1993; Egendorf 1985; Gibbs 1989; Kinzie 1989; Mahedy 1986; North et al. 1989; Obenchain and Silver 1992; Wilson 1989). This recognition has coincided with national discussions of a spiritual approach to health and healing and with the inclusion in DSM-IV of a new, nonpathological category, "religious or spiritual problem," within the subsection titled "Other Conditions That May Be a Focus of Clinical Attention." (American Psychiatric Association 1994; Van Biema 1996; Wallis 1996).

In recent decades, psychotherapeutic emphasis has moved from classic psychodynamic conflicts over sexual and aggressive strivings toward a focus on self-affirmation and on existential issues that have been raised in connection with 20th-century wars and calamities. It has been observed that this century has witnessed vast gains in scientific understanding without concomitant advances in spiritual awareness. In other words, great scientific breakthroughs have left us with more knowledge but perhaps less peace (Epstein 1995). In this chapter we explore the relationships between traumatic events and moral, spiritual, and religious issues. Our examination of the distinction between spirituality and religion is undertaken with full realization of the multiplicity of religious and spiritual backgrounds present in our pluralistic culture.

Moral Crisis

One therapist put it this way: "We aren't just counselors, we're almost priests. They come to us for absolution as well as help" (Marin 1981, p. 68). In two seminal articles, Peter Marin (1980, 1981) described individual "moral pain" after war-related trauma. Marin observed that one of the great American therapeutic dreams is that the past is escapable, that suffering can be avoided, that happiness is always possible, and that insight inevitably leads to joy. Life's lessons, however, teach us something else again, because the past pursues those who have been traumatized. "The closer they come to the truth of their acts," said Marin (1981, p. 74), "the more troubled they are, the more apart they find themselves and the more tragic becomes their view of life."

In describing Vietnam veterans' war guilt, Marin (1981) pointed to Karl Jasper's use of the term *metaphysical guilt*, which has to do with the relationship of humankind to God and the ways in which the human race has somehow betrayed its given covenant with God. Interpreting Jasper's meaning, Marin explained that this guilt refers to a collective failure to extend our own sense of human reciprocity or responsibility past our own family and/or nation to include those unlike ourselves. In this context, each individual is answerable both to his or her own conscience and to God, and individuals remain responsible for setting right what they themselves perceive to be wrong.

Marin's views set the stage for renewed interest in and commentary about spiritual aspects of PTSD. Most mental health workers would acknowledge that people who are truly traumatized undergo a deep moral crisis that may be the first step in a lifelong struggle to reconstitute values, beliefs, and a sense of meaning in life. Indeed, a traumatic experience may be some individuals' first encounter with evil. They may realize that they have committed, or been victims of, acts with real and terrible consequences that have shattered their sense of an understandable reality (Marin 1981). Three assumptions may be destroyed by these experiences: 1) the belief in one's personal invulnerability, 2) the perception of the world as comprehensible, and 3) the view of oneself in a positive light (Janoff-Bulman 1985). Once basic assumptions are challenged, there is a universal need to make sense of what has happened. A rupture of trust in oneself, in one's assessment of reality, and in one's simple sense of competence occurs (Stone 1992). When death, destruction, and survival are confluent, there may be a premature encounter with mortality (Jacob 1987).

Many combat veterans assumed that having survived the war meant that their dues had been paid and their personal struggles were over. They subsequently discovered that this was not the case—that until their experiences were placed into a meaningful perspective, reevaluated, and then described to friends and family at home, their journey was incomplete. Moreover, many Vietnam veterans, influenced by the antiwar movement, interpreted their wartime experience as negative, which led to further reluctance to integrate these experiences into their lives (Tice 1996). Not only did individual victims and healers fail to entirely understand the scope of the effect of traumatization, but often the environment failed to empathically respond to traumatized individuals (Brett 1993). Furthermore, it has been empirically demonstrated that PTSD among Vietnam combat veterans carries a considerable risk for suicide and that intensive combat-related guilt is the most significant explanatory factor (Hendin and Haas 1991).

Nevertheless, in the aftermath of even the most bitter, cynical, and angry psychological responses to trauma, most traumatized individuals desperately seek some sort of insight or proof that meaningful life is possible. Regardless of whether symptoms of pathology appear, a trauma survivor will often focus more attention on a quest for meaning and a search for purpose than on superficial pursuits (Decker 1993). Ritual and ceremony provide one way of returning to a civilized life and achieving control of one's destiny. Although they will never be entirely free of symptoms, survivors understand that ritual facilitates grieving by providing an opportunity to face memories of the war in a constructive environment (e.g., the Vietnam Veterans' Memorial in Washington, D.C.) and that healing must come from within. The search for meaning and the moral dilemmas engendered by trauma ultimately motivate individuals to seek answers that will enable them to resolve the conflicts created by their experience.

Religion

The trauma survivor's quest for meaning and purpose frequently begins with religion. As our discussion in the previous section implied, traumatic experiences provoke fundamental questions about good, evil, and the deeper meaning of an individual's life. Even more importantly, these experiences raise the issue of whether a human being's existence, once transformed by devastating personal experience, can be restored to wholeness.

Raising these questions brings one face to face with an even larger and more profound set of questions. What exists over and beyond the Self? Nothing? Something? If there is something existent beyond the Self, what are Its nature and characteristics? Does It exist over and above everything else, or can It be subjugated to other realities? Does It have the power to change reality? Is Its power benign and life-creating or malignant and life-destroying? What function does It have in a person's traumatic experience? What function, if any, can It have in the healing and restoration to wholeness of someone who has been traumatized?

Religion posits a particular set of systematized answers to such existential questions. This systemization creates a framework of explanatory symbols and concepts (i.e., theology) that can be employed to interpret and understand life experience. From this explanatory framework evolves the ritual, communal structure, and sacred writings that we associate with institutionalized religion (see Chapter 2 in this volume). The principle of trust in, and surrender to, the will of the Deity as a means of resolving and transforming life crises is a major teaching of most world religions(see Chapter 1 in this volume).

Judaism holds open the possibility of being restored to a right relationship with God through atonement. In ancient Judaism, specific sacrifices were prescribed by the Law to atone for sin. In contemporary Judaism, Yom Kippur (the Day of Atonement) serves the same purpose. Christianity teaches that repentance for sin, accompanied by turning to God and asking to be united with the atoning sacrifice of Christ, brings forgiveness and the gift of new life. Christian trauma survivors often list "the loss of God" as one of their greatest privations (Tice 1996, p. 2). Buddhists believe in accepting life as it comes, including traumatic events. They follow the teachings of the prophet Buddha, who found freedom from the bondage of riches and power through surrender to a new life of service to the poor. Reincarnation is a major tenet of the Buddhist faith. Buddhists believe in Karma (merit), the notion that a person's actions in this life will affect the kind of existence he or she will have in the next (Epstein 1995).

The Cambodians who suffered severe upheaval and traumatization during the Pol Pot era of 1975–1979 are predominantly Buddhist. Coexisting with traditional Buddhist doctrine in Cambodia are traditional folk religions that incorporate a variety of animistic, ancestral, or ghostlike spirits. In the wake of trauma, the belief that the spirits of the deceased continue to be present has at times been known to provide more comfort than some traditional Buddhist tenets (Boehnlein 1987). Both folk and traditional religions require performance of certain rituals as means of coping with despair and unhappiness (Kinzie 1989).

Most Eastern religions include the belief that one's existence does not cease upon physical death. Consequently, those who expect that their Karma future will result in a positive outcome may anticipate death less fearfully death. Within the Hindu theory of transmigration, for example, the soul is believed to pass through a series of births, and existence is only one manifestation of universal animation. As a result, devout Hindus are more likely to "surrender" to the inevitableness of life, including death (Brende 1993).

Aspects of the religious belief systems of Native Americans have been incorporated successfully into a healing program—the sweat lodge ceremony—that has been used to treat combat-related PTSD. Usually led by a tribal medicine man, this ceremony is essentially a purification rite in which participants' warrior identities are transformed into a more nurturing and mature form of adaptation. The ritual helps male warriors to reaffirm a sense of connectedness to society (Silver and Wilson 1988; Wilson 1989). A key component is the involvement of both combat and noncombat members of the veterans' community (Obenchain and Silver 1992).

Attempts to include some form of spiritual/religious development in Western psychological descriptions of health have ranged from the early Freudian perspective of religion as a prerational infantile state developed to cope with individual psychological instincts to more contemporary transpersonal descriptions of spiritual/mystical pursuits as essential and present in all aspects of human life. Most psychological descriptions of spiritual growth and identity indicate spiritual discovery results in a change in personality toward greater harmony, altruism, resourcefulness, integration, and other generally desirable qualities (Decker 1993).

Some people, however, find organized religion to be an unsatisfactory resource for dealing with questions of meaning and a search for purpose in life. Moreover, many Vietnam veterans identify organized religion with the "establishment" they feel has betrayed them. Others find organized religion to be more concerned with superficial matters of institutional maintenance than with the search for life's purpose. Referring individuals with PTSD to a religious institution to assist them in their quest for meaning may not be universally effective. The quest may be more successful in a therapeutic setting. If posttraumatic moral and spiritual issues are to be therapeutically addressed, it is important to understand some of the spiritual dynamics of PTSD.

Spirituality

Although no single definition of the concept exists, spirituality has been described as "the transcendental relationship between the person and a Higher Being, a quality that goes beyond a specific religious affiliation . . . " (Peterson and Nelson 1987, p. 35). Whereas spirituality is essentially a subjective sacred experience, religion involves subscribing to a set of beliefs or doctrines that have been institutionalized. In this context, spirituality is not limited to any one set of doctrines or practices. From a psychological perspective, spirituality is a universal experience, not a universal theology (Vaughn 1991). Historically, spirituality was not widely distinguished from religion until the rise of secularism in the 20th century, when some people became disillusioned with religious institutions, seeing them as preventing rather than facilitating a personal transcendent experience (Turner et al. 1995).

In the past 25 years, the split between religion and spirituality has led to the widespread development of spiritual practices not associated with recognized religious institutions. Although confidence in religion and religious leadership may be decreasing, the number of people who report that they believe in God or some spiritual force, who pray or engage in some spiritual practice, and/or who report religious or mystical experiences has remained constant or has slightly increased (Jones 1993; Lukoff et al. 1992). The trend toward secularization "has not created an irreligious culture, only an unchurched one" (Stark and Bainbridge 1985, p. 441). Accordingly, it is not surprising that human reactions to overwhelming stress should involve spiritual elements.

Mythic Systems

Human beings have a central core of emotions, thoughts, reality perceptions, and memories that forms identity and awareness. In theological language, this central core is the soul (or, in Greek, *psyche)*. Spirituality refers to the relationship between this central core, or psyche, and ultimate eternal reality (or, in more direct terms, the relationship between the soul and God). The desire to be spiritual leads people to form an identification with a mythic system (Fergueson 1995).

Mythic systems are composed of three elements: 1) a symbolic narrative that portrays the relationship between the individual and ultimate eternal transcendent reality (e.g., the Gospels, Vision Quest stories), 2) a system of rituals used to unite the individual with the ultimate eternal transcendent reality, and 3) interpretive concepts (theology) that define and explain the spiritual. These concepts are used to interpret human experience in the context of the symbolic narrative (i.e., they give meaning to life experience). Mythic systems often become formalized and institutionalized into religions (Fergueson 1995).

The process of identification with a mythic system begins early in life. In America, even families without a formal religious affiliation often encourage their children to identify with some mythic system. In other words, children are encouraged to be spiritual. Because of early identification, a mythic system may be a person's only available source for interpreting life experience. When traumatic stress elicits profound spiritual questions about good, evil, right, wrong, and the meaning of human existence, people naturally turn to their identified mythic system to find answers. With some investigative encouragement, people with PTSD may describe mythic interpretations of their traumatic experience (Fergueson 1995).

This spiritual context is important and in some cases may be crucial, as the following example illustrates.

> A few years ago, one of the authors (JFF) was invited to talk to a Vietnam veteran who was being treated in a Veterans Administration outpatient clinic. He encountered a man in a deep state of anxiety and agitation. During the interview, the man wrung his hands so violently that he abraded the skin. The man told him about what he had done in Vietnam. He also reported that he had recently prayed for the recovery of his critically ill lover and had promised God that if she recovered he would give up drugs. Although she recuperated, he was unable to give up his addiction and subsequently developed an extreme case of agoraphobia. When the author explored why the veteran was frightened to leave home, he said, "You ought to know. You're a priest. You know that I'm a double sinner. God is going to kill me!" His identified mythic system taught him that to breach a promise to God meant inevitable destruction.
>
> The author had only a short time with the man but tried to introduce some alternative ideas. He attempted to present a view of God as loving, creative, and forgiving. The initial goal was to liberalize the man's identified mythic system by suggesting that other mythic ideas could be equally true. The author reminded the veteran about the biblical statement "God is love." How could the One who is "love" be bent upon destroying a person's life? Why would Jesus forgive sinners if God was ultimately going to destroy them for their transgressions? The veteran's regular therapist volunteered to continue the process of helping the patient form a more constructive identification.

In this example, the spiritual context of PTSD was key to understanding this veteran's acute anxiety. Sometimes, as therapists wrestle unconsciously with the enormity of their patients' experiences, they rediscover mythic stories (Lindy 1989; Shay 1994). As they do so, therapists begin to understand more and patients begin to feel understood.

Evil

Individuals are often uncomfortable with the supernatural dualistic conceptualizations of evil that are frequently encountered in religious circles. Evil exists as something intrinsic to human experience. There has been philosophical and theological debate about whether evil exists as a separate force (out there) or whether it exists only in the hearts of humans (Prins 1994). Whatever its origin, evil is a force "that seeks to kill life and liveliness" (Peck 1988, p. 43), often through powerful acts of aggression employed to control, dominate, or manipulate. The cumulative force of such actions is so potent as to be perceived as a supernatural, transcendent experience more powerful than oneself, because the self cannot control or defend against it. In other words, people who have been traumatized to the degree that they manifest PTSD often have had a watershed ecstatic transcendent encounter with evil. The affective component of this encounter often correlates with descriptions of mystical experiences.

Over the past 7 years, one of the authors (JFF) has worked with dozens of Vietnam veterans and abuse survivors who have had spiritual issues connected with trauma. Characteristically, most of these individuals have identified with mythic systems that assume an absolute split between good and evil (or perceive evil as distinct from good). Simply stated, good is always good. Evil is always evil. Good is never evil. Evil is never good. Prior to their traumatic experience, these individuals' spiritual identification was solely with good. However, in their traumatic experience, they either acted in ways they perceived to be evil or were victims of evil actions. Because of the absolute split between good and evil in their mythic systems, they believe that their encounter with evil has permanently defiled them and made them children of evil, who deserve nothing but evil, and who will never be good again. Ultimately, these individuals have no sense of difference between good and evil. Unfortunately, many of them have never revealed these feelings and ideas to their therapists—or if they have, they have been rebuffed.

> One veteran told his therapist that he was "Satan's child" because of his war experiences. The therapist explained to the veteran that this was an irrational and superstitious idea that was being used to avoid responsibility. Although the therapist's explanation may have had intellectual merit, it overlooked the personal impact of the man's encounter with evil and his mythic identification. Calling himself "Satan's child" was, in part, a way of understanding and giving meaning to his experience. The veteran abandoned therapy because he felt the therapist had discounted his ideas.

Ecstatic Experience

There is a correlation between the affective state experienced in deep prayer and the depersonalization and derealization encountered in the dissociative episodes that are occasionally part of PTSD. Dissociative experiences of being "outside of the body" or being suspended in peacefulness mirror the contemplative states of Christian mystics.

In the language of spirituality, the depersonalization and derealization common to mystical experience are called *ecstasy*. The word ecstasy comes from the Greek *ek-stasis*, which means "to be placed outside" (Liddell and Scott 1953). An ecstatic experience places one outside normal reality. According to the *Oxford Dictionary of the Christian Church* (Cross 1966), the chief characteristic of the ecstatic state is the "alienation of the senses. The body, unable to bear the strain, becomes usually unmovable, and sight, hearing, etc., cease to function" (p. 437). The DSM-IV description of depersonalization disorder states that

> [t]here may be a sensation of being an outside observer of one's mental processes, one's body, or parts of one's body. Various types of sensory anesthesia, lack of affective response, and a sensation of lacking control of one's actions, including speech, are often present." (American Psychiatric Association 1994, p. 488)

There is thus a similarity between spiritual descriptions of ecstasy and psychological descriptions of depersonalization. Traumatized people experiencing dissociation may be undergoing, in spiritual terms, an ecstatic experience. Individuals may perceive dissociation positively or negatively. The spiritual power and magnitude of the experience derive from a sense of being placed outside normal reality.

Dissociation is often the result of being overwhelmed by forces that are stronger than the ego's defense mechanisms—a condition that serves to reinforce the spiritual power and importance of the dissociative episode. People who undergo severe trauma may experience dissociation as an ecstatic spiritual process that allows them to mentally remove themselves from the situation. In times of crisis and instability, individuals often turn to such a powerful source of psychic energy to restore and stabilize the psyche. For example, individuals under stress may try to reexperience a dissociative state in an attempt to gain distance from the intensity of their emotions.

Reenactment

Individuals with PTSD are drawn to reenact, either directly or symbolically, their traumatic experience, particularly during times of high stress. This drive makes sense in the spiritual context of PTSD. Reenactment involves *ritual-*

ized patterns (i.e., doing things in a specific, repetitive manner) that in theological language could be called *action*. Often accompanying this repetitive action are duplications of thought and language that in theological terminology could be considered *form*. Frequently, objects, dress, and/or location are used repeatedly; such elements could theologically be termed *matter*.

Action, form, and matter are the hallmarks of worship. The Christian sacrament of the Holy Eucharist (i.e., Communion or the Lord's Supper) provides a useful illustration. The *matter* of the sacrament consists of the bread and wine. The *form* of the sacrament is composed of the words spoken during consecration of the bread and wine. The *action* is the ceremonial process of taking, blessing, breaking, and distributing the bread and wine (Cross 1966). Worshipers participating in this sacrament are reenacting the sacrifice of Jesus in order to receive psychic energy.

Worship is used to unite people with transcendent reality so that the power of that reality can be made apparent to them. In spiritual terms, people who are reenacting a traumatic experience are engaging in worship. Application of the theological categories of action, matter, and form to reenactment episodes reveals striking similarities with more customary forms of worship.

Last year, a psychiatrist friend said, in exasperation, in reference to one of his PTSD patients, "She seems to worship her trauma." He was correct. People trust their experience. The most powerful ecstatic transcendent experience of his patient's life was connected with her trauma. Whenever she reached a crisis point, she reenacted. Although her response seems inappropriate, the trauma survivor who reenacts is no different from the parishioner who lights votive candles and attends daily Mass during a personal crisis. Both are illustrations of worship designed to connect a person with an external transcendent source of psychic power. The problem is that the psychiatrist's patient is essentially worshiping something that is ultimately destructive. The spiritual task for this patient is to experientially discover a transcendent source of psychic energy that is life-giving, healing, and restorative.

In working with PTSD patients, we have discovered that they are reluctant to give up a transcendent source of power, no matter how destructive, until they have had enough consistent experience with another source to be able to trust it.

A counselee of one of the authors (JFF), a young woman with an extensive history of childhood sexual abuse, continually reenacted her trauma by engaging in abusive sexual encounters during times of personal crisis. The author provided her with a supply of consecrated communion wafers and encouraged her to receive communion whenever she felt compelled to reenact. For 6 months, she experimented with either communion or reenactment when under stress. At the end of the 6 months, receiving communion replaced reenactment. The woman stated that she had made the behavioral change because " . . . it works. Communion gives me strength. I don't hurt myself when I receive communion."

In order to have a complete patient profile, it is important for the therapist to examine what is actually occurring in the spiritual context of a person's life, rather than simply relying on that person's verbal reports. People may turn to religion in the aftermath of trauma in an effort to heal themselves. Although their language may indicate that spiritual change is taking place in their lives, in times of stress and crisis, they may regress and reenact their traumatic experience. The essential problem for the therapist attempting to help such individuals then becomes determining whether they are truly learning to accept a new source of transcendent energy that is both healing and restorative.

Conclusions

There is a spiritual context in PTSD treatment. Most traumatized people had a mythic system identification in place prior to their traumatic experience. Exploring that system can loosen sticking points that impede therapeutic progress. Stress powerful enough to produce PTSD involves profound spiritual dynamics that may hold a person captive to the traumatic experience. Awareness can open new avenues for both healing and restoration and can also provide a helpful model for comprehending resistance to PTSD treatment.
    Robert Bly (1990) has written that

> . . . where a man's wound is, that is where his genius will be. Wherever the wound appears in our psyches, whether from an alcoholic father, shaming mother, shaming father, abusing mother, whether it stems from isolation, disability or disease, that is precisely the place from which we will give our major gift to the community. (p. 42)

To complete the journey, to heal both self and community, the traumatized person must return to society as a witness. "I access my experience in healing from trauma to assist others in their journey home. My work is exactly where my wound is." (Tice 1996, p. 3). Ultimately, the process is a redemptive one. The challenge to our humanity is there, yet so is the opportunity to understand our dark side, to overcome and be true to ourselves. To make use of this opportunity may be to embrace grace.

References

American Psychiatric Association: Diagnostic and Statistical Manual of Mental Disorders, 3rd Edition. Washington, DC, American Psychiatric Association, 1980

American Psychiatric Association: Diagnostic and Statistical Manual of Mental Disorders, 3rd Edition, Revised. Washington, DC, American Psychiatric Association, 1987

American Psychiatric Association: Diagnostic and Statistical Manual of Mental Disorders, 4th Edition. Washington, DC, American Psychiatric Association, 1994

Bly R: Iron John. Reading, MA, Addison Wesley, 1990

Boehnlein JK: Clinical relevance of grief and mourning among Cambodian refugees. Soc Sci Med 25:765–772, 1987

Brende JO: A 12-step recovery program for victims of traumatic events, in International Handbook of Traumatic Stress Syndromes. Edited by Wilson JP, Raphael B. New York, Plenum, 1993, pp 867–877

Brett EB: Psychoanalytic contributions to a theory of traumatic stress, in International Handbook of Traumatic Stress Syndromes. Edited by Wilson JP, Raphael B. New York, Plenum, 1993, pp 61–68

Carmil D, Breznitz S: Personal trauma and world-view—are extremely stressful experiences related to political attitudes, religious beliefs, and future orientation? J Trauma Stress 4:393–405, 1991

Cross FL (ed): The Oxford Dictionary of the Christian Church. London, Oxford University Press, 1966

Decker LR: The role of trauma in spiritual development. J Humanistic Psychology 33(4):33–46, 1993

Egendorf A: Healing From the War. Boston, MA, Houghton Mifflin, 1985

Epstein M: Thoughts Without a Thinker: Psychotherapy From a Buddhist Perspective. New York, Basic Books, 1995

Fergueson JF: The spiritual context of PTSD (abstract). Presentation as part of an Issue Workshop ("Reassessing PTSD: Spiritual and Sociopolitical Contexts") at the Annual Meeting of the American Psychiatric Association, Miami, FL, May 1995

Gibbs MS: Factors in the victim that mediate between disaster and psychopathology. J Trauma Stress 2:489–513, 1989

Hendin H, Haas AP: Suicide and guilt as manifestations of PTSD in Vietnam combat veterans. Am J Psychiatry 148:586–591, 1991

Horowitz MJ: Stress-response syndromes: a review of post-traumatic stress and adjustment disorders, in International Handbook of Traumatic Stress Syndromes. Edited by Wilson JP, Raphael B. New York, Plenum, 1993, pp 49–60

Jacob MR: A pastoral response to the troubled Vietnam veteran, in Post-Traumatic Stress Disorders: A Handbook for Clinicians. Edited by Williams T. Cincinnati, OH, Disabled American Veterans National Headquarters, 1987, pp 51–74

Janoff-Bulman R: The aftermath of victimization: rebuilding shattered assumptions, in Trauma and Its Wake, Vol 1. Edited by Figley CR. New York, Brunner/Mazel, 1985, pp 15–35

Jones JW: Living on the boundary between psychology and religion. Psychol Religion Newslett 18(4):1–7, 1993

Kinzie JB: Therapeutic approaches to traumatized Cambodian refugees. J Trauma Stress 2:75–95, 1989

Liddell HG, Scott R: A Lexicon Abridged From Liddell and Scott's Greek–English Lexicon. London, Oxford University Press, 1953

Lindy JD: Transference and post-traumatic stress disorder. J Am Acad Psychoanal 17:397–413, 1989

Lukoff D, Lu F, Turner R: Toward a more culturally sensitive DSM-IV: psycho-religious and psychospiritual problems. J Nerv Ment Dis 180:673–682, 1992

Mahedy WP: Out of the Night. New York, Ballantine, 1986

Marin P: Coming to terms with Vietnam. Harper's 261(12):41–56, 1980

Marin P: Living in moral pain. Psychology Today 6(11):68–74, 1981

North CS, Smith EM, McCool RE, et al: Acute postdisaster coping and adjustment. J Trauma Stress 2:353–360, 1989

Obenchain JV, Silver SM: Symbolic recognition: ceremony in a treatment of post-traumatic stress disorder. J Trauma Stress 5:37–43, 1992

Peck MS: People of the Lie: The Hope for Healing Human Evil. London, Rider, 1988

Peterson EA, Nelson K: How to meet your clients' spiritual needs. J Psychosoc Nurs Ment Health Serv 25:34–39, 1987

Prins H: Psychiatry and the concept of evil. Br J Psychiatry 165:297–302, 1994

Shay J: Achilles in Vietnam: Combat Trauma and the Undoing of Character. New York, Atheneum, 1994

Silver SM, Wilson JP: Native American healing and purification rituals for war stress, in Human Adaptation to Extreme Stress From the Holocaust to Vietnam. Edited by Wilson JP, Harel Z, Kahan B. New York, Plenum, 1988, pp 337–355

Sparr LF: Post-traumatic stress disorder: does it exist? Neurol Clin 13(2):413–429, 1995

Stark R, Bainbridge WS: The Future of Religion. Berkeley, CA, University of California Press, 1985

Stone AM: The role of shame in post-traumatic stress disorder. Am J Orthopsychiatry 62:131–136, 1992

Tice SN: From trauma to enlightenment: the survivor's journey. Post-Traumatic Gazette 1(5):2–3, 1996

Turner RP, Lukoff D, Barnhouse RT, et al: Religious or spiritual problem: a culturally sensitive diagnostic category in the DSM-IV. J Nerv Ment Dis 183:435–444, 1995

Van Biema D: Emperor of the soul. Time 147(26):65–68, 1996

Vaughn F: Spiritual issues in psychotherapy. J Transpers Psychol 23(2):105–119, 1991

Wallis C: Faith and healing. Time 147(26):59–62, 1996

Wilson JP: Trauma, Transformation and Healing. New York, Brunner/Mazel, 1989

ᥫᩣ CHAPTER 7 ᥫᩣ

The Role of Clergy in Mental Health Care

David B. Larson, M.D., M.S.P.H.,
Mary Greenwold Milano, B.A.,
Andrew J. Weaver, M.Th., Ph.D., and
Michael E. McCullough, Ph.D.

In this chapter we outline the relationships that exist among clergy, mental health professionals, and mental health patients. We also offer suggestions for building more constructive relationships among clergy, mental health professionals, and mental health patients as we approach the 21st century. To begin to understand the current nature of these relationships, it is important to consider research on 1) the religious life of Americans; 2) the roles that religious practices, beliefs, and values may play in the prevention of mental health problems; and 3) how religious commitment may influence patients' decisions about mental health care.

———
Preparation of this manuscript was supported by the generosity of the John M. Templeton Foundation and King Pharmaceuticals, a division of Monarch Pharmaceuticals.

Research Findings on Religion and Mental Health

Numerous national surveys have established the central role of religion in the lives of many Americans. As an example, nearly 95% of Americans report a belief in God, 57% report praying daily, and 42% report having attended church in the past week (Princeton Religion Research Center 1994). These religious beliefs also seem to play a critical role in many Americans' decision-making processes; almost three-quarters of Americans say that their approach to life is grounded in their religious beliefs (Bergin and Jensen 1990).

Americans' religious beliefs appear to be quite relevant in the mental health arena. Indeed, Lukoff et al. (1992) stated that "the religious and spiritual dimensions of culture are among the most important factors that structure human experience, beliefs, values, behavior, and illness patterns" (p. 673). To illustrate, research has shown that patients' religious beliefs can influence their thoughts about the etiology of their illness; many psychiatric patients believe that their illness is a punishment from God or the result of personal wrongdoing or sin (Bearon and Koenig 1990; Sheehan and Kroll 1990). In fact, a national survey of psychologists found that nearly two-thirds of patients used religious language during treatment to express their problems and conflicts (Shafranske and Malony 1990).

Other studies have found that higher levels of religious commitment are associated with enhanced feelings of well-being and a lower prevalence of mental illness. For example, several studies have found that the religiously committed enjoy a greater sense of overall life satisfaction (Hadaway and Roof 1978; Poloma and Pendleton 1990), as well as lower rates of depression (Hertsgaard and Light 1984; Mayo et al. 1969; McClure and Loden 1982), compared with the nonreligious. Religion has also been identified as a potential buffer against stress; the religiously committed report lower stress levels, adjust better to stress, and experience fewer adverse consequences of stress than do the less committed (Lindenthal et al. 1970; Stark 1971; Williams et al. 1991).

Religious commitment may also potentially play a role in reducing suicide rates (Agnew 1998; Weaver and Koenig 1996). A systematic review of published studies evaluating religion's influence on suicide rates found that religious commitment was associated with lowered suicide rates in nearly every study (Gartner et al. 1991). Indeed, non–church attenders have been found to be four times more likely to commit suicide than frequent church attenders (Comstock and Partridge 1972), and lack of or infrequent attendance at religious worship services has been identified as an important—although frequently overlooked—predictor of suicide (Stack 1983).

Religion may serve as a potential deterrent not only to suicide but also to other self-destructive behaviors, such as drug and alcohol abuse. Indeed, the presence of religion in an individual's life seems to be linked with a decreased risk of drug abuse. Several studies have identified religious commitment as a variable that is consistently and negatively associated with tobacco, alcohol, and illicit-drug use (Gartner et al. 1991; Hays et al. 1986; Oleckno and Blacconiere 1991). Gorsuch and Butler (1976) were one of the first to comment on the predominantly negative relationship between religious commitment and drug abuse:

> Whenever religion is used in an analysis, it predicts those who have not used an illicit drug regardless of whether the religious variable is defined in terms of membership, active participation, religious upbringing, or the meaningfulness of religion as viewed by the person himself. (p. 127)

More recent research has established a significant relationship between religious commitment and nonuse (or moderate use) of alcohol (Cochran et al. 1988). Most interestingly, regardless of whether a religion specifically proscribed or preached/warned against alcohol use, individuals who were active in a religious congregation consumed substantially less alcohol than did those who were not active (Amoateng and Bahr 1986). Similarly, a national survey of 12,000 adolescents documented that the lowest rates of adolescent drug abuse were found among the more theologically conservative religious groups, and that even the more theologically liberal groups still had slightly lower rates of drug abuse than did the nonreligious (Loch and Hughes 1985). In addition, the researchers found that of all the various single-item measures of religious commitment employed, the item "importance of religion" was the best predictor of the absence of substance abuse.

Although much of the research on religion and mental health has focused on prevention, a growing body of literature has begun to suggest that religion may also be associated with more rapid clinical improvement or enhanced mental health care outcomes. In the early 1970s, Andreasen (1972) heralded the potentially beneficial clinical role that a religious perspective can play in helping individuals cope with and recover from depression. More recent studies have supported the finding that religion is associated with an improvement in overall emotional functioning. For example, previously hospitalized schizophrenia patients who attended church or who received supportive aftercare from religious caregivers were found to have lower overall rates of rehospitalization (Chu and Klein 1985; Katkin et al. 1975). In addition, following participation in religious worship, a significant reduction in numbers of psychiatric symptoms has been noted both on patient self-report measures and on more objective measures such as electromyelogram (EMG) biofeedback (Elkins et al. 1979; Finney and Malony 1985; Griffith et al. 1986; Morris 1982). Some studies have even suggested that treatment for religious patients is most effective when it incorporates elements of the patient's own religious belief system (Propst 1980; Propst et al. 1992).

Given the demonstrated personal importance, as well as clinical relevance, of religion for many Americans, it is not surprising that many patients desire to have their religious orientations and belief systems taken into account during their health care and treatment. Surveys have found that more than 75% of respondents believe that physicians should address spiritual issues as part of the medical care, and about 40% actively want such patient–provider dialogue to take place (D. E. King and Bushwick 1994; Maugans and Wadland 1981). Even more surprisingly, nearly half of patients want their physicians to pray with them (D. E. King and Bushwick 1994). The need to address patients' spiritual issues is particularly salient in the mental health setting, where treatment approaches inevitably touch on intensely personal issues, including worldviews, values, and beliefs (Bergin 1980).

The Role of Clergy in Mental Health Treatment

Care Provided by Hospital Chaplains

Given the importance of religious and spiritual perspectives to patients when they are facing illness or distress, clergy are in a unique position to support and complement traditional medical care (McSherry et al. 1986). For example, Florell (1973) found that orthopedic patients who received supportive and informative visits from clergy while in the hospital recovered more quickly from surgery, had lower levels of surgery anxiety, and made fewer requests for hospital services than did patients who were not visited by clergy. The author noted that "the implication of this for hospital administration is obvious in terms of bed availability, physician time, cost, and patient satisfaction" (Florell 1973, p. 35). Other studies have reported beneficial effects from hospital-based pastoral care intervention; these results have included increased patient satisfaction (Parkum 1985), increased medical knowledge and treatment compliance (Saunders and Kong 1983), and overall decreased rates of hospitalization (Tubesing et al. 1977).

In addition, hospital-based clergy seem to be more highly regarded by patients than are other nonmedical support services within the hospital setting. When VandeCreek et al. (1991) compared patients' attitudes toward chaplains, social workers, and patient representatives, they found that patients rated chaplains as providing more important services and meeting their needs more effectively than the other two nonmedical services studied. In fact, from a hospital administrative perspective, patients who felt that clergy met their needs for counseling and support during their hospital stay were more likely to select that hospital again and recommend it to others. Findings such as these have led some researchers to comment that "chaplaincy could perform in the hospital setting as a legitimate clinical service to the spiritual (motivation, values, meaning, and belief) dimension of the patient to show how critical full, healthy functioning of this dimension is to rapid and full patient recovery" (McSherry and Nelson 1987, p. 210).

Clergy as Initial Mental Health Providers

Not only do clergy provide needed support to frontline medical providers, but they are also often called upon to act as frontline mental health providers themselves. A 20-year study on the patterns of emotional help–seeking in the United States reported that about 40% of Americans seek out a member of the clergy when dealing with a personal problem (Veroff et al. 1981). Among people who attended religious services at least once per week, more than 50% considered clergy to be their primary mental health care providers. Surprisingly, even among those individuals who were not religiously active and who described themselves as seldom attending religious services, 16% reported seeking out clergy for help with personal problems. These findings led the researchers to comment that "one cannot fail to be impressed by the continuing role that clergy play in assisting many Americans in dealing with personal problems" (Veroff et al. 1981, p. 134).

Weaver (1995) commented on the counseling practices of the clergy, noting that

[a]ccording to the United States Department of Labor, there are approximately 312,000 Jewish and Christian clergy serving congregations in America . . . engaged in mental health counseling at the rate of 7 hours per week, with an additional 2.5 hours per week in supportive mental health services. This totals 148.2 millions hours of mental health services. The mental health services provided by these clergy is equivalent to each of the 77,000 associate and full-time members of the American Psychological Association delivering services at the rate of 38.5 hours per week. This estimate does not take into ac-

count the nearly 100,000 nuns in full-time religious vocation in the Catholic Church or clergy from other religious traditions in the United States, about whom it appears we have no research data regarding counseling knowledge or activity. (p. 132)

Not only are Americans turning to clergy in large numbers for initial help, but they also seem to be highly satisfied with the quality of care that they are receiving. A comprehensive survey of Americans who sought outside help for personal problems showed that 58% felt that they were "helped" or "helped a lot" by their visits to a member of the clergy, whereas only 11% believed that their experience with clergy "did not help" (Veroff et al. 1981). These percentages compare favorably with ratings of psychologists and psychiatrists, who were described by 62% of individuals as having "helped" or "helped a lot," whereas 20% claimed that their experience with mental health professionals "did not help." Clergy also were rated more highly than mental health professionals on several interpersonal traits, such as warmth, caring, stability, and—somewhat surprisingly—professionalism (Schindler et al. 1987).

Despite these substantial numbers, research is needed to assess clergy effectiveness. As yet, there are few studies that assess the effectiveness of clergy-provided mental health care (Arnold and Schick 1979; Worthington 1986; Worthington et al. 1996?]). Given this lack of demonstrated effectiveness, why are Americans turning to the clergy for help in such large numbers? First, the American public is highly religious, and numerous researchers have commented that some patients may prefer obtaining assistance from an individual who shares their fundamental belief system (R. R. King 1978; Larson et al. 1986; Maugans and Wadland 1981; Propst et al. 1992; Richards and Davison 1989). These findings have been supported by a national survey that found that two-thirds of the general population "would prefer a counselor who is religious" (Ross 1993). Indeed, for the more than 70% of the population for whom religious commitment is a central life theme, therapeutic methods that ignore this religious belief system " . . . may provide an alien values framework. . . . A majority of the population probably prefers an orientation . . . that is sympathetic, or at least sensitive to, a spiritual perspective" (Bergin and Jensen 1990, p. 6).

Why might patients prefer a therapist who shares or values their religious and spiritual beliefs? This proclivity to prefer providers whose belief systems are tolerant toward or similar to their own could be motivated by patients' fears of having their beliefs misunderstood or even belittled (American Psychiatric Association 1990). Keating and Fretz (1990) found that religiously committed patients did have more reservations about therapy, including fears that the therapist would ignore their spiritual concerns, view their religious or spiritual beliefs as pathological or bizarre, reject the idea of communicating with a higher power, or assume that they shared the therapist's own (probably nonreligious) belief system. In fact, patient–provider religious value differences can cause therapeutic difficulties. Research has demonstrated that patients whose values deviate from those of their therapist are more likely to receive a poor prognosis than patients whose values are more similar to those of their therapist (Kelly and Strupp 1992; Szasz 1970).

Some patients may even fear that the therapist might try to change their religious or spiritual views or beliefs. Indeed, research has identified a large divergence between patients' and mental health professionals' religious and spiritual beliefs (Bergin and Jensen 1990; Henry et al. 1971; Larson et al. 1986). Although few studies have investigated this phenomenon, results reported in one study, an analysis of patients' assimilation of their therapist's overall value systems (Kelly and Strupp 1992), suggest that fears of troubling clinical outcomes may be unfounded. These authors found that whereas most patients' values moved closer toward those of the therapist, patients' religious values showed little or no change or movement toward the therapist's religious or spiritual values.

If 40% of Americans turn to clergy as their initial or primary mental health resource, regardless of the reasons behind this choice, what types of disorders are clergy encountering? Several studies have shown that clergy are frontline mental health workers not just for individuals with minor adjustment disorders, but also for those with serious mental disorders. In a survey of more than 200 members of the clergy conducted in Connecticut by Mollica et al. (1986), 85% reported having counseled dangerous or suicidal individuals, and a full 100% stated that they had provided some type of crisis intervention for their clients. Building on the finding that clergy were a significant mental health resource for troubled individuals, Larson et al. (1988) analyzed data from the five-site Epidemiologic Catchment Area (ECA) survey sample of more than 18,000 adults. They found that individuals with serious psychiatric illnesses (e.g., major depression, schizophrenia, panic attacks, manic depressive disorder) were just as likely to seek treatment from a clergy member as from a mental health professional.

Educational Preparation and Efficacy of Pastoral Counselors

If clergy are seeing and treating people with serious mental disorders, how well prepared are they for the task of providing effective assessment and care?

Not very well prepared, according to the available body of research on the subject. Domino (1990) found that a representative sample of Catholic, Protestant, and Jewish clergy demonstrated about the same level of knowledge about symptoms of emotional distress as did a group of college students in an introductory psychology class. Other researchers have noted that clergy score significantly lower than professionally trained mental health providers such as psychologists, psychiatrists, social workers, and marriage and family therapists on their ability to assess an individual's suicide potential (Holmes and Howard 1980).

Even clergy themselves seem to recognize their deficiencies in handling mental health issues. When Weaver (1995) examined 14 years' worth of published research concerning the clergy, he found that between 50% and 80% of clergy in the reviewed studies considered their seminary training in pastoral counseling to be deficient and reported feeling inadequately prepared to deal with the serious psychiatric and marital problems to which they were frequently being asked to respond. Another survey of nearly 2,000 Methodist pastors found that whereas nearly 95% believed that having counseling training in seminary was important, only 25% of pastors felt that their seminary training had contributed significantly to their competence in pastoral counseling (Orthner 1986). In fact, nearly 40% of pastors surveyed agreed that the overall quality of pastoral counseling is inadequate.

Quality seminary education on mental health issues or counseling techniques does seem to be conspicuously lacking. Linebaugh and Devivo (1981) surveyed 55 accredited Protestant seminaries in the United States and found that nearly one-half had no course requirements in the area of pastoral care or counseling. Even though most of the seminaries contacted in the study indicated that their students not only were aware of the need for counseling courses but also were actively seeking to take such courses, the majority of seminaries had no clear consensus on what required courses or even electives should make up such an educational track.

Fostering and Improving Dialogue Between Religious and Mental Health Professionals

It is not in the best interests of our patients that 1) most clergy recognize that counseling individuals is important yet report that they have not obtained the necessary training to do so effectively, and 2) the majority of mental health professionals recognize that an understanding of religious issues is important to their patients yet admit that they are not adequately trained in handling religious issues in clinical care (see Chapter 9 in this volume). One can only be left with the impression that clergy and mental health professionals are singing the same song, only different verses. If mental health professionals are trained in counseling techniques but not in religious aspects of care, and if clergy are trained in religious aspects of care but not in counseling techniques, would not these complementary educational inequities provide a near-perfect opportunity for each side to begin to support and complement the other's continuing and recognized deficiencies?

Unfortunately, until recently, religiously committed patients have had difficulty finding mental health providers who were both competent to treat a wide range of psychiatric problems and respectful of (and conversant in relevant aspects of) their patients' religious commitments. Patients are left with the following dilemma: Should they, on the one hand, seek out a mental health professional and hope that their religious beliefs will not be ridiculed or labeled as "neurotic," pathological, or even psychotic (Ellis 1988; Freud 1930/1961; Group for the Advancement of Psychiatry 1976; Horton 1974; Mandel 1980)? Or should they instead opt for a clergy member or pastoral counselor who will deal sensitively with their religious beliefs but perhaps lack the necessary clinical expertise required to treat their psychiatric problem?

We posit that members of the religious sector as well as the mental health community bear equal responsibility in continuing the (in essence) de facto separation between "the couch and the cloth" (Larson et al. 1988). Despite research suggesting that up to one-third of the individuals counseled by clergy may have severe mental illness (Pattison 1969), clergy refer less than 10% of their clients to mental health professionals (Lee 1976; Mollica et al. 1986; Piedmont 1968; Virkler 1979). Likewise, even though clinicians are frequently unprepared and usually untrained to deal with the spiritual issues that 75% of patients (according to research estimates) are bringing up during their medical care or psychotherapy, mental health professionals seem to be even less likely than clergy to cross-refer their patients (Gottlieb and Olfson 1987; Larson et al. 1988; Mollica et al. 1986).

Fortunately, recent clinical and policy decisions by governing organizations within the mental health field have begun to open the door to further dialogue between the religious and mental health professional sectors, enriching treatment options for patients—particularly religiously or spiritually committed patients. What steps have been taken by the mental health field to try to incorporate spiritual sensitivity into clinical treatment? One of the first major steps toward the recognition and acceptance of religious and spiritual factors in the therapeutic setting occurred as recently as 1990, when the

American Psychiatric Association's (APA) Board of Trustees issued an official action titled "Guidelines Regarding Possible Conflict Between Psychiatrists' Religious Commitments and Psychiatric Practice." These groundbreaking directives advised the psychiatric community that "it is useful for clinicians to obtain information on the religious or ideological orientation and beliefs of their patients so that they may properly attend to them in the course of treatment" (American Psychiatric Association 1990). For the first time, religion and spirituality were professionally recognized as not just acceptable but important treatment factors—a substantial policy shift from traditionally held positions in the psychiatric community that assumed religious or spiritual commitment to be irrelevant or even pathological (Larson et al. 1992, 1993).

Just as the APA's official action statement opened the door to enhancing religious sensitivity in the clinical setting, so, too, did the fourth edition of the *Diagnostic and Statistical Manual of Mental Disorders* (DSM-IV; American Psychiatric Association 1994) lay the foundations for religious sensitivity in the diagnostic process. In response to the publication of several articles noting examples of DSM-III-R's (American Psychiatric Association 1987) negative bias toward religion (Larson et al. 1993; Lukoff et al. 1992; Post 1992; Richardson 1993), sections containing insensitive representations of religious or spiritual experiences were eliminated in DSM-IV. In addition, a new category, "religious or spiritual problem," was added to the V codes (i.e., conditions not attributable to a mental disorder) in the DSM-IV section titled "Other Conditions That May Be a Focus of Clinical Attention." Lukoff et al. (1992) described this new V code category in their article on psychiatry's need for increased cultural sensitivity in handling clinical issues related to religion and spirituality:

> *Psychoreligious* problems are experiences that a person finds troubling or distressing and that involve the beliefs and practices of an organized church or religious institution. Examples include loss or questioning of a firmly held faith, change in denominational membership, conversion to a new faith, and intensification of adherence to religious practices and orthodoxy.
>
> *Psychospiritual* problems are experiences that a person finds troubling or distressing that involve that person's reported relationship with a transcendent being or force. These problems are not necessarily related to the beliefs and practices of an organized church or religious institution. Examples include near-death experience and mystical experience. This [V code] category can be used when the focus of treatment is a psychoreligious or psychospiritual problem that is not attributable to a mental disorder. (pp. 676–677)

Building Collaborative and Mutual Learning Relationships Between Religious and Mental Health Professionals

If mental health professionals are being encouraged to recognize and deal more sensitively with religious and spiritual issues in treatment, yet lack the ability to do so, how can needed changes be accomplished? We suggest that clergy can begin to facilitate this learning process by stepping out of their traditional supportive and clerical roles into a more specific educational role in regard to mental health professionals. If mental health professionals have opened the door to religion, then clergy could be seen as having the responsibility to respond to this collaborative opportunity. In turn, mental health professionals need to learn to use the expertise of clergy more effectively in the clinical setting and to refer patients to clergy when appropriate—in short, to regard clergy as knowledgeable and relevant sources of information for learning to deal sensitively with patients' religious issues.

There are numerous ways in which this collaborative and mutual learning relationship can begin to develop. Excellent resources have recently become available that can help to provide guidance in this learning process. For example, in response to the recent mandate for psychiatric residency training programs to include training on religious and spiritual sensitivity in clinical care, a group of psychiatrists have published "A Model Curriculum for Psychiatry Residency Training Programs: Religion and Spirituality in Clinical Practice" (Larson et al. 1996). This document not only provides educational models for structured core and accessory lectures on religion and spirituality in the psychiatric setting but also suggests ways in which psychiatry residents and pastoral care professionals can learn together. For example, hospital chaplains can be invited to take the now-mandated religion and psychiatry course with psychiatric residents. By mixing clergy and residents together in the same learning format, clergy can learn more about psychiatric approaches to illness, and residents can begin to let go of preconceived notions about the role of the clergy in medicine and learn to see them as valuable contributors to the medical process. In addition, this learning format allows clergy and residents to discuss ways in which referrals between clergy and mental health professionals would be helpful for enhancing patients' treatment outcomes. Such a process opens up lines of communication between medical professionals and clergy, making it easier and more natural for young mental health professionals to consult with clergy later in their careers.

Another avenue for fostering collaborative and mutual learning relationships between the two professions involves the use of community clergy as guest lecturers on the belief systems of the major world religions. This approach helps to break down religious stereotypes that may be held by faculty or residents and opens up the possibility of using skilled clergy as consultants on cases with particularly problematic or difficult-to-manage religious content. Clergy members could also be invited to participate in discussions of cases involving religious or spiritual issues. This format allows for cross-disciplinary discussion and furthers mental health professionals' understanding of normative religious beliefs and practices (versus abnormal beliefs or practices that may signal underlying psychopathology). Such an approach also helps to solidify mental health professionals' perceptions of clergy as professionals and provides them with a better understanding of how clergy can assist them in clinical assessment, care, and treatment. In addition, clergy are exposed to the intricacies of psychiatric treatment, making them more educated collaborators and fostering a better understanding of current psychiatric practices and approaches.

Residents can increase their effectiveness by meeting with the chaplain assigned to the inpatient ward at the beginning of their inpatient assignments to determine what services the chaplain may be able to offer patients and ward staff. Such an interaction can establish a precedent as well as an expectation that each newly assigned resident might interact and collaborate with the chaplain at an initial point in his or her rotation. Residents could even be required to refer at least one very religious inpatient to the chaplain for pastoral care or for the completion of a religious history to further their knowledge of clerical resources.

Of course, if mental health professionals are willing to begin collaborating with clergy and other pastoral care professionals, clergy or chaplains must take responsibility for making this interaction clinically productive. If clergy who participate in case conferences or courses have negative attitudes toward psychiatry, are overly defensive about their religious teachings, or use their participation in the educational process as an opportunity to proselytize, they may reinforce mental health professionals' negative opinions about interfacing or collaborating with the clergy. In addition, clergy or chaplains may vary considerably in their clinical and educational abilities, residents' experiences with them may not be uniformly constructive or educationally beneficial. As a result, medical faculty must use discretion when selecting which clergy members to invite to participate in case conferences or courses, and they may need to follow up with these religious professionals to provide constructive feedback on recent presentations in order to improve future collaborative efforts. Clergy need to be receptive to such feedback and learn to tailor their messages to medical professionals.

Clinical professionals frequently look to unbiased, objective resources such as research findings to assess the merits of undertaking new clinical collaborative efforts, such as interfacing with clergy. Unfortunately, clergy are at a distinct disadvantage in this regard, given the extreme paucity of published research on the effectiveness of pastoral interventions. Some hospital administrators may seek to limit the role of chaplains within the hospital setting, and without credible, empirical research documenting their effectiveness, chaplains may have little recourse. The new guidelines for residency training programs, which mandate the inclusion of material on the clinical relevance of religious issues to mental health treatment and diagnosis, do provide an opening for clergy, but outcome research is desperately needed to bolster the case that psychiatric patients' religious beliefs are indeed clinically relevant and that pastoral services are an essential resource for addressing important patient needs.

The religious and pastoral care community cannot afford to maintain the status quo regarding the lack of published research data on pastoral interventions by allowing this gap in the literature to continue (Larson et al. 1995). Chaplains and clergy should endeavor to collaborate on research teams within the hospital or university setting, where they can lobby to include religious measures or considerations into new mental health research initiatives. In so doing, they will be helping to build upon the ever-growing but still limited body of research on religion and mental health, as well as to legitimize their role in the mental health care delivery process.

Increasing collaboration between mental health professionals and clergy is not an easy task. There has been a history of misunderstanding, suspicion, and distrust between these groups. However, as the impact that religion can have on mental health status and the importance of handling religious issues sensitively in treatment continue to move into the forefront of mental health discourse, both groups must take steps to close the gulf that has long separated them. Through open dialogue, structured clinical interactions, and the growing body of empirical literature, both mental health professionals and clergy can provide those suffering from mental health problems with the psychiatrically balanced and spiritually integrated help that they seek but do not always find.

References

Agnew R: The approval of suicide: a social-psychological model. Suicide Life Threat Behav 28:205–225, 1998

American Psychiatric Association: Diagnostic and Statistical Manual of Mental Disorders, 3rd Edition, Revised. Washington, DC, American Psychiatric Association, 1987

American Psychiatric Association: Guidelines regarding possible conflict between psychiatrists' religious commitments and psychiatric practice. Am J Psychiatry 147:542, 1990

American Psychiatric Association: Diagnostic and Statistical Manual of Mental Disorders, 4th Edition. Washington, DC, American Psychiatric Association, 1994

Amoateng AY, Bahr SJ: Religion, family, and adolescent drug use. Sociological Perspectives 29:53–73, 1986

Andreasen NJ: The role of religion in depression. Journal of Religion and Health 11:153–166, 1972

Arnold JD, Schick C: Counseling by clergy: a review of empirical research. Journal of Pastoral Counseling 14:76–101, 1979

Bearon LB, Koenig HG: Religious cognitions and use of prayer in health and illness. Gerontologist 30:249–253, 1990

Bergin AE: Psychotherapy and religious values. J Consult Clin Psychol 48:95–105, 1980

Bergin AE, Jensen JP: Religiosity of psychotherapists: a national survey. Psychotherapy 27:3–7, 1990

Chu C, Klein HE: Psychological and environmental variables in outcome of black schizophrenics. J Natl Med Assoc 77:793–796, 1985

Cochran JK, Begley L, Bock EW: Religiosity and alcohol behavior: an exploration of reference group therapy. Sociological Forum 3:256–276, 1988

Comstock GW, Partridge KB: Church attendance and health. Journal of Chronic Diseases 25:665–672, 1972

Domino G: Clergy's knowledge of psychopathology. Journal of Psychology and Theology 18:32–39, 1990

Elkins D, Anchor KN, Sandler HM: Relaxation training and prayer behavior as tension reduction techniques. Behavioral Engineering 5:81–87, 1979

Ellis A: Is religiosity pathological? Free Inquiry 8(2):27–32, 1988

Finney JR, Malony HN: An empirical study of contemplative prayer as an adjunct to psychotherapy. Journal of Psychology and Theology 13:284–290, 1985

Florell J: Crisis intervention in orthopedic surgery—empirical evidence of the effectiveness of a chaplain working with surgery patients. Bulletin of the American Protestant Hospital Association 37:29–36, 1973

Freud S: Civilization and its discontents (1930), in Standard Edition of the Complete Psychological Works of Sigmund Freud, Vol 21. Translated and edited by Strachey J. London, Hogarth, 1961, pp 59–145

Gartner J, Larson DB, Allen GD, et al: Religious commitment and mental health: a review of the empirical literature. Journal of Psychology and Theology 19:6–25, 1991

Gorsuch RL, Butler MC: Initial drug abuse: a view of predisposing social psychological factors. Psychol Bull 3:120–137, 1976

Gottlieb JF, Olfson M: Current referral practices of mental health care providers. Hospital and Community Psychiatry 38:1171–1181, 1987

Griffith EE, Mahy GE, Young JL: Psychological benefits of spiritual Baptist "mourning," II: an empirical assessment. Am J Psychiatry 143:226–229, 1986

Group for the Advancement of Psychiatry: Mysticism: Spiritual Quest or Mental Disorder? New York, Group for the Advancement of Psychiatry, 1976

Hadaway CK, Roof WC: Religious commitment and the quality of life in American society. Review of Religious Research 19:295–307, 1978

Hays RD, Stacy AW, Widaman DMR, et al: Multistage path models of adolescent alcohol and drug use: a reanalysis. Journal of Drug Issues 16:357–369, 1986

Henry WE, Sims JH, Spray SL: The Fifth Profession: Becoming a Psychotherapist. San Francisco, CA, Jossey-Bass, 1971

Hertsgaard D, Light H: Anxiety, depression, and hostility in rural women. Psychol Rep 55:673–674, 1984

Holmes CB, Howard ME: Recognition of suicide lethality factors by physicians, mental health professionals, ministers, and college students. J Consult Clin Psychol 48:383–387, 1980

Horton PC: The mystical experience: substance of an illusion? J Am Psychoanal Assoc 22(1–2):364–380, 1974

Katkin S, Zimmerman V, Rosenthal J, et al: Using volunteer therapists to reduce hospital readmissions. Hospital and Community Psychiatry 26:151–153, 1975

Keating AM, Fretz BR: Christians' anticipations about counselors in response to counselor descriptions. Journal of Counseling Psychology 37:293–296, 1990

Kelly TA, Strupp HH: Patient and therapist values in psychotherapy: perceived changes, assimilation, similarity, and outcome. J Consult Clin Psychol 60:34–40, 1992

King DE, Bushwick B: Beliefs and attitudes of hospital inpatients about faith healing and prayer. J Fam Pract 39:349–352, 1994

King RR: Evangelical Christians and professional counseling: a conflict of values. Journal of Psychology and Theology 6:276–281, 1978

Larson DB, Pattison EM, Blazer DG, et al: Systematic analysis of research on religious variables in four major psychiatric journals: 1978–1982. Am J Psychiatry 143:329–334, 1986

Larson DB, Hohmann AA, Kessler LG, et al: The couch and the cloth: the need for linkage. Hospital and Community Psychiatry 39:1064–1069, 1988

Larson DB, Sherrill KA, Lyons JS, et al: Associations between dimensions of religious commitment and mental health reported in *American Journal of Psychiatry* and *Archives of General Psychiatry*: 1978–1989. Am J Psychiatry 149:557–559, 1992

Larson DB, Thielman SB, Greenwold MA, et al: Religious content in the DSM-III-R glossary of technical terms. Am J Psychiatry 150:1884–1885, 1993

Larson DB, Greenwold MA, Brown D, et al: Mental health and religion, in The Encyclopedia of Bioethics. Edited by Reich WT, Post SG. New York, Macmillan, 1995, pp 1704–1711

Larson DB, Lu FG, Swyers JP: A Model Curriculum for Psychiatry Residency Training Programs: Religion and Spirituality in Clinical Practice. Rockville, MD, National Institute for Healthcare Research, 1996

Lee RR: Referral as an act of pastoral care. Journal of Pastoral Care 30:186–197, 1976

Lindenthal JJ, Myers JK, Pepper MK, et al: Mental status and religious behavior. Journal for the Scientific Study of Religion 9:143–149, 1970

Linebaugh DE, Devivo P: The growing emphasis on training pastor–counselors in Protestant seminaries. Journal of Psychology and Theology 9:266–268, 1981

Loch BR, Hughes RH: Religion and youth substance abuse. Journal of Religion and Health 24:197–208, 1985

Lukoff D, Lu F, Turner R: Toward a more culturally sensitive DSM-IV: psychoreligious and psychospiritual problems. J Nerv Ment Dis 180:673–682, 1992

Mandel AJ: Toward a psychobiology of transcendence: God in the brain, in The Psychobiology of Consciousness. Edited by Davidson RJ, Davidson JM. New York, Plenum, 1980

Maugans TA, Wadland WC: Religion and family medicine: a survey of physicians and patients. J Fam Pract 23:210–213, 1981

Mayo CC, Puryear HP, Richeck HG: MMPI correlates of religiousness in late adolescent college students. J Nerv Ment Dis 149:381–385, 1969

McClure RF, Loden M: Religious activity, denomination membership, and life satisfaction. Psychology, A Quarterly Journal of Human Behavior 19:13–17, 1982

McSherry E, Nelson WA: The DRG era: a major opportunity for increased pastoral care impact or a crisis for survival? Journal of Pastoral Care 41:210–211, 1987

McSherry E, Kratz D, Nelson W: Pastoral care departments: more necessary in the DRG era? Health Care Manage Rev 11:47–59, 1986

Mollica RF, Streets FJ, Boscarino J, et al: A community study of formal pastoral counseling activities of the clergy. Am J Psychiatry 143:323–328, 1986

Morris PA: The effect of pilgrimage on anxiety, depression, and religious attitude. Psychol Med 12:291–294, 1982

Oleckno WA, Blacconiere MA: Relationship of religiosity to wellness and other health related behaviors and outcomes. Psychol Rep 68:819–826, 1991

Orthner DK: Pastoral Counseling: Caring and Caregivers in the United Methodist Church. Nashville, TN, General Board of the Higher Education and Ministry of the United Methodist Church, 1986

Parkum K: The impact of chaplaincy services in selected hospitals in the eastern United States. Journal of Pastoral Care 39:262–269, 1985

Pattison EM: The role of clergymen in community mental health programs. International Psychiatry Clinics 5:245–256, 1969

Piedmont EB: Referrals and reciprocity: psychiatrists, general practitioners, and clergymen. J Health Soc Behav 9:29–41, 1968

Poloma MM, Pendleton BF: Religious domains and general well being. Social Indicators Research 22:255–276, 1990

Post SG: DSM-III-R and religion. Soc Sci Med 35:81–90, 1992

Princeton Religion Research Center: Religion in America, 1993–1994. Princeton, NJ, Princeton Religion Research Center, 1994

Propst RL: The comparative efficacy of religious and nonreligious imagery for the treatment of mild depression in religious individuals. Cognitive Therapy and Research 4:167–178, 1980

Propst RL, Ostrom R, Watkins P, et al: Comparative efficacy of religious and nonreligious cognitive-behavioral therapy for the treatment of clinical depression in religious individuals. J Consult Clin Psychol 60:94–103, 1992

Richards PS, Davison ML: The effects of theistic and atheistic counselor values on client's trust: a multi-dimensional scaling analysis. Counseling and Values 33: 109–120, 1989

Richardson JT: Religiosity as deviance: negative religious bias in and misuse of the DSM-III. Deviant Behavior: An Interdisciplinary Journal 14:1–21, 1993

Ross RJ: Future of pastoral counseling: legal and financial concerns, in The Future of Pastoral Counseling: Whom, How and For What Do We Train? Edited by McHolland J. Fairfax, VA, American Association of Pastoral Counselors, 1993, p 115

Saunders T, Kong W: The role for churches in hypertension management. Urban Health 12:49–51, 1983

Schindler F, Barren MR, Hannah MT, et al: How the public perceives psychiatrists, psychologists, nonpsychiatric physicians, and members of the clergy. Professional Psychology: Research and Practice 18:371–376, 1987

Shafranske EP, Malony HN: Clinical psychologists' religious and spiritual orientations and their practice of psychotherapy. Psychotherapy 27:72–78, 1990

Sheehan W, Kroll J: Psychiatric patients' belief in general health factors and sin as causes of illness. Am J Psychiatry 147:112–113, 1990

Stack S: The effect of the decline in institutionalized religion on suicide: 1954–1978. Journal for the Scientific Study of Religion 22:239–252, 1983

Stark R: Psychopathology and religious commitment. Review of Religious Research 12:165–176, 1971

Szasz T: The Manufacturer of Madness: A Comparative Study of the Inquisition and the Mental Health Movement. New York, Harper & Row, 1970

Tubesing DA, Holinger PC, Westberg GE, et al: The Wholistic Health Center Project: an action-research model for providing preventive, whole person health care at the primary level. Med Care 15:217–227, 1977

VandeCreek L, Jessen A, Thomas J, et al: Patient and family perceptions of hospital chaplains. Hospital and Health Services Administration 36:455–467, 1991

Veroff J, Kulka RA, Douvan E: Mental Health in America: Patterns of Help Seeking From 1957 to 1976. New York, Basic Books, 1981

Virkler HA: Counseling demands, procedures, and preparation of parish ministers: a descriptive study. Journal of Psychology and Theology 7:271–280, 1979

Weaver AJ: Has there been a failure to prepare and support parish based clergy in their role as frontline community mental health workers? A review. Journal of Pastoral Care 49:129–148, 1995

Weaver AJ, Koenig HG: Elderly suicide, mental health professionals, and the clergy: a need for clinical collaboration, training, and research. Death Studies 20:495–508, 1996

Williams DR, Larson DB, Buckler RE, et al: Religion and psychological distress in a community sample. Soc Sci Med 32:1257–1262, 1991

Worthington EL Jr: Religious counseling: a review of published empirical research. Journal of Counseling and Development 64:421–431, 1986

Worthington EL, Kurusu TA, McCullough ME, et al: Empirical research on religion and psychotherapeutic processes and outcomes: a ten-year review and research prospectus. Psychol Bull 119:448–487, 1996

SECTION III

❧

Looking Toward the Future

ᕲᕲ CHAPTER 8 ᕲᕲ

The Worlds of Religion and Psychiatry

Bioethics as Arbiter of Mutual Respect

Laurence J. O'Connell, Ph.D., S.T.D.

"War of the Worlds!" Orson Welles, in his 1938 broadcast, alarmed a large segment of the American population by announcing that aliens from another planet were invading Planet Earth. The reaction of the radio audience that evening highlighted a common human trait: flight in the face of the unknown and rejection on the basis of difference. Cultural anthropology provides ample empirical evidence of our innate standoffishness and tendency to view those people different from us as "other." We are most comfortable within prescribed boundaries and familiar surroundings. Xenophobia crisscrosses the history of humanity.

Xenophobia is not confined to the grand stage of nationalistic and tribal politics; it spills over into the everyday life and common experience of individuals and communities. Whether we express it through such sinister forms as racial and gender discrimination or through the relatively innocent fervor of the sports fanatic, we commonly exclude foreign ranges of experience from our purview. For example, many commentators have insisted that science and religion are incompatible worlds, categorically distinct and mutually exclusive. In 1984, the National Academy of Sciences insisted on this chasm:

"Religion and science are separate and mutually exclusive realms of human thought whose presentation in the same context leads to misunderstanding of both scientific theory and religious belief" (Jones 1994, p. 186).

This insistence on separating science and religion, coupled with Freud's notoriously negative view of religion, has influenced psychiatry, which "in its diagnosis classification systems as well as its theory, research, and practice has tended to either ignore or pathologize the religious and spiritual dimensions of life" (Lukoff et al. 1992, p. 673). Although historically there have always been those like William James and Carl Gustav Jung who readily acknowledged common ground with religion, psychotherapists have only gradually warmed to the notion that the religious dimension of human existence may be directly relevant to the success of their own practice (Jones 1994, p. 18). Today, though, we do find representatives of both religion and psychiatry "searching for public philosophies that will overcome the estrangement between them" (Wind 1990, p. 89). There seems to be a mutual readiness to acknowledge that religion is more than a primitive psychological mechanism, on the one hand, and that psychiatry need not seek to replace religion, on the other. In short, religion can be partner to psychiatry and psychiatry need not be religion's predator. This chapter represents a modest contribution to forging a basic understanding that could allow religion and psychiatry to relate more easily and productively.

A rapprochement between religion and psychiatry would most likely benefit both therapists and their patients as well as pastoral counselors and their clients. It is important, however, to clearly differentiate the respective domains of religion and psychiatry and to establish an ethically informed perspective that will help span these different worlds while respecting the integrity of each. Absent such distinction and perspective, misunderstanding is indeed likely. Fortunately, tools are available for this task. Phenomenology, for example, provides a suitable method for distinguishing between the respective worlds of religion and science, while bioethics provides an appropriate framework for exploring the moral parameters of their relationship.

William James and the Phenomenological Method

William James is probably best known for his *Principles of Psychology* (1890/1950) and his *Varieties of Religious Experience* (1902/1963). In *Principles* James laid out the world in psychological terms, while in *Varieties* he expounded his view of the religious propensities of human nature. The preeminent contribution of William James to the worlds of psychology and religion, though, is not found solely in these classic works. A thorough study of his writings reveals that James had captured, although in an inchoate way, the essence of what would become known as phenomenology. In fact, the acknowledged founder of the phenomenological movement, Edmund Husserl, studied William James and viewed him as a great genius. Much to Husserl's chagrin, James did not reciprocate his adulation, dismissing Husserl as an obscure German metaphysician.

It is fitting that the incipient phenomenology of William James, America's first professor of psychology, provides the foundation for drawing necessary distinctions between the realms of psychiatric and religious practice. Although he never systematically applied his seminal phenomenological insights to building connections between psychology and religion, James did resist the dichotomizing and dismissive tendencies of many of his contemporaries. For example, he held that the psychophysical conditions, healthy or morbid, attendant upon the genesis of any experience—including religious experience—say nothing with regard to the significance or value of that experience. "There is not a single one of our states of mind, high or low, . . . that has not some organic process as its condition" (James 1902/1963, p. 281). Thus, it is not exceptional to think that "every religious phenomenon has its history in and its derivation from natural antecedents" (James 1902/1963, p. 281). Here James was explicitly refuting those who theorized that religion was perverted sexuality, an aberration of the digestive system, or some other dysfunction.

In rebutting "the bugaboo of morbid origin" (James 1902/1963, p. 284) of religious experience, James' forward-looking approach allowed for the potential human and spiritual value of religious phenomena, but it did little to explain their essential nature and inner dynamics. Here James' incipient phenomenology proves instructive. It yields a basic understanding of religious consciousness while establishing the grounds for distinguishing religious experience from other realms of human experience. Moreover, in describing how different realms of experience relate to one another, James' phenomenology legitimates active dialogue and encourages a balanced relationship between religion and psychiatry.

James' phenomenological perspective encompasses two important points that are relevant to this discussion, namely, the *intentionality of consciousness* and the notion of *multiple realities*. This is not the place to discuss in detail these complicated and sophisticated philosophical ideas, but a brief overview of each will give us what we need in the context of bioethics.

Intentionality of Consciousness

The contention that consciousness is intentional is rooted in the view that knowledge is more than a simple relatedness to an object. Knowing is "an active and in fact creative achievement, rather than a passive or merely static directedness" (Spiegelberg 1969, p. 116). James saw "the goal of the mind as 'to take cognizance of a reality, *intend it*, or be "about" it' " (Spiegelberg 1969, p. 116). In short, James stressed the *subjective* dimension of experience by insisting that we make a substantial contribution to the shape of our own experience. James did not exclude attention to the objective or to behavior by any means, but he insisted that the subject cannot be viewed "as absolutely passive clay, upon which 'experience' rains down" (James 1902/1963, p. 521). James frankly stated that the origin "of all reality, whether from the absolute or the practical point of view, is subjective, is ourselves" (James 1890/1950, p. 491). We always interpret our surroundings; there is indeed a "world out there," but our knowledge of it is never passive perception, never pure and simple. The experiencing subject is not "simply a passive recipient of the data presented. . . . There is actually no completely passive subject" (Smith 1966, p. 521). That which is experienced is inextricably related to the experient, and it is this bipolarity that constitutes the universe of experience and the foundation of the reality we know.

The intentionality of consciousness, which highlights the subjective sources of cognition, is central to the phenomenological approach. It is no surprise, then, that phenomenologists are not primarily concerned with the ontological status of the objects they study. Rather, phenomenologists are "interested in their *meaning*, as it is constituted by the activities of the mind" (Schutz 1941, p. 115). For example, the fact that the unicorn reportedly grazing in the park might not really exist "out there" is not particularly important to the phenomenologist *as* phenomenologist. Although the unicorn may not roam about in the town square, it does inhabit the world of myth. What *is* important is that the unicorn, as object of mythology, is constituted or has validity through specific acts of consciousness—that is, mythic consciousness, which is governed by its own rules of internal consistency. It is the essential conditions of the unicorn as *meant* (intended) that lie at the heart of phenomenological inquiry. In other words, phenomenology focuses on the meaning of an object rather than its place in the material world. Phenomenology helps explain how the same thing can carry different meanings, how one person's serene mystical revelation, for example, is experienced by another person as a frenzied psychotic episode. The subjective character of intentional consciousness implies that the world can be engaged in many different ways.

Multiple Realities

Raw perceptual experience, that ill-defined and inarticulate world within reach of our senses, is the subjective foundation of everything we count as real, according to James.

> The 'paramount reality' is given to us through our *perceptual* insertion among other beings and objects in whom we have a practical and emotional involvement through our 'tangible' relationships with them. It can be defined as . . . the world we can grasp immediately, upon which we can act and which can act upon us. (Edie 1970, p. 238)

We work within the world of immediate perceptual experience to construct the contours and content of a meaningful existence. We organize and shape our everyday world. Yet, the paramount reality of the ordinary world of perception in which we live our everyday lives is not as monolithic as it usually seems.

Although he considered the world of ordinary perception or the sphere of practical realities as "paramount reality," James also recognized that there are "many worlds" or "subuniverses" of reality that surround and are founded on the structures of the perceptual world. James held that several—or, more likely, an infinite number of—"subuniverses" or various orders of reality exist, each characterized by its own special and separate style of existence. Each subuniverse is a world unto itself, and "each world, while it is *attended to*, is real after its own fashion" (James 1890/1950, p. 293). We are, for example, *really* terrified at the approach of a knife-wielding assailant, and we cry out, until we are awakened and reassured that it was just a dream. Yet, we still tremble and feel that something really did happen. And it did! The reality of the dream world only loses its hold on us when we are somehow shaken or shocked back into the world of ordinary perception. Reality, then, is "an analogous term which we predicate in different ways, depending on the various 'subuniverses' to which we refer a given experience" (Stephens 1974, p. 111). This is another way of stating that consciousness is intentional—that is, that meaning is constituted in the activities of the mind or that "consciousness can live in different orders of reality" (Edie 1969, p. 92)

Although the most fundamental modality of intentional experience is perceptual, there are other modes of intentional consciousness that give us access to what might be called subsidiary orders of reality—the realms of imagination and recollection, for instance. Husserl referred to these subsidiary orders of reality as "quasi-worlds" or "different fields of presence" (Husserl 1939/1973, pp. 171, 181), while the renowned phenomenologist

Alfred Schutz adopted the term "finite provinces of meaning." They are finite because the meaning(s) that reside in each are limited to that specific sphere of consciousness. An atheist, for example, is impervious to the presence or reality of God because the atheist has not entered into the specifically religious province of meaning. So, when Catholics speak of the real presence of Jesus Christ, atheists predictably respond with disbelief. They cannot "get into it." God is most emphatically not real! In other words, they simply cannot constitute meaning for themselves in religious terms, although they may well do so in the future. Religious conversion involves entering what Husserl called "a different field of presence" where God becomes *real* and available to the believer, but this move cannot be forced, since "we cannot create belief out of whole cloth when our perception actively assures us of its opposite" (James 1902/1963, p. 214).

James' phenomenological insight led him to conclude that "the whole distinction of real and unreal, and the whole psychology of belief, disbelief, and doubt, are grounded on two mental facts—first, that each of us is liable to think differently of the same; and second, that when we have done so, we can choose which way of thinking to adhere to and which to disregard" (James 1890/1950, p. 290). Belief in God, for example, can go either way. Fields of presence, subuniverses of reality, provinces of meaning are either constituted or dissolved through acts of intentional consciousness. A former believer, for instance, might say that she has lost her faith in the existence of God. Put somewhat differently, the reality of God has evaporated for someone who has "lost the faith." That particular province of meaning is simply no longer accessible.

Religious Consciousness and Psychic Reality: Worlds Apart

The phenomenological theories of intentionality of consciousness and multiple realities provide the critical insights we need to differentiate between the worlds of psychiatry and religion. Although both religion and psychiatry are among those weasel words that are capable of many twistings and turnings, it is possible to distinguish their respective foci and special interests.

Again, William James gives practical guidance by providing a serviceable definition of religion: The religious province of meaning comprises the experiences of individuals "so far as they apprehend themselves to stand in relation to whatever they may consider the divine" (James 1902/1963, p. 50).

Religious consciousness repositions the self in relation to a divine mystery and constitutes "an absolute addition to the Subject's range of life" (James 1902/1963, p. 64). It gives the believer "a new sphere [or province] of power" that provides stability, continuity, consolation, and strength for dealing with life's challenges and contingencies—illness, death, evil, personal tragedy. For the believer, religious consciousness is the center of dynamic energy, "the hot place in a man's consciousness, the group of ideas to which he devotes himself, and from which he works, call it *the habitual center of his personal energy*" (James 1902/1963, p. 200).

Psychiatry deals with the study, diagnosis, treatment, and prevention of mental disorders. These disorders present mainly with disturbances of emotion, thought, perception, and behavior, and they are often not readily traceable to identifiable physical causes. Psychiatrist Patrick Staunton made the following point:

> Psychiatry, as a branch of medicine, is dedicated to diagnosing and treating disease whenever possible, using scientifically based knowledge, but always aims at comforting the sick and alleviating suffering. Unlike general medicine, psychiatry is a service profession dedicated to care for the sick even in the absence of scientifically based knowledge of the sickness. (McCarthy 1990, p. 41)

Psychiatry, then, operates within specific provinces of meaning, namely, the "particularized fabrics of disordered personhood" (Wallace 1994, p. 86). The mental and emotional disorders and behavioral dysfunctions that psychiatry confronts emanate from "hot spots" within the intentional consciousness of individuals. These hot spots become the habitual center of personal energy that exhibit themselves in personal neurotic symptom formation or character pathology. In cases of serious mental illness "the person is generally unaware that he is ill (he 'loses insight')" (Gelder 1986, p. 1147). In the vocabulary we have been developing here, persons move into finite provinces of private meaning that, sadly, they may never escape. The mentally ill are often trapped within closed provinces of meaning where they coexist with alien realities that remain inaccessible to others. The fabric of their disordered personhood is so tightly woven as to be impermeable.

Religion and psychiatry focus on different finite provinces of meaning that exhibit different constituent elements. Religious consciousness moves away from self and toward the Other. It engenders a range of experience that elicits "a feeling of being in a wider life than that of this world's selfish little interests; and a conviction, not merely intellectual, but as it were sensible, of the existence of an Ideal Power" (James 1902/1963, p. 269). Religious consciousness constitutes a constructive, positive, and socially engaged attitude toward life.

By contrast, psychiatry addresses forms of consciousness, ranges of experience that are inherently disordered, often generating disturbed and negative personal and social orientations. In attending to "highly particularized fabrics of disordered personhood," psychiatry deals with the psychotic and maladaptive aspects of isolated individual life. This is not to say that psychiatry is indifferent to the social ramifications of disturbed individual behavior. It is rather that its primary point of departure, although not its exclusive concern, is the individual.

In some very definite ways, then, religion and psychiatry are worlds apart. They operate within the purview of independent and irreducible provinces of meaning, each characterized by its own special and separate style of existence. An authentic object of religious experience cannot inhabit psychotic consciousness, and vice versa. For example, a mystical experience that is authentically religious cannot at the same time be a psychotic episode. And conversely, a genuinely psychotic state cannot be authentically religious. In other words, "there is no possibility of referring one of these provinces to the other by introducing a formula of transformation" (Schutz 1941, p. 232). There are no hybrids here.

Religion and Psychiatry: Adjacent Planes, Likely Partners

The French have a wonderful and, in this particular context, very applicable phrase: *degagement pour engagement* ("disengage to engage"). It is often necessary and certainly always wise to elucidate specific differences before naively suggesting the terms of any relationship. In carefully delimiting the respective worlds of religion and psychiatry, we have exposed the anatomy of difference. And we must insist on certain absolute distinctions. Yet, psychiatry and religion often move in similar regions of interest and inquiry that require engagement and cooperation.

For instance, religious language and behavior can be mimicked in mental illness. "There is no doubt that psychiatric illness can manifest itself in religious expression," so the potential for confusing or mislabeling the distinct provinces of religion and mental illness is quite possible (Post 1992, p. 87). W. W. Meissner (1991) explains that to the extent that a patient uses religious beliefs to prevent or subvert effective and adaptive functioning or as an expression of personality disturbance or symptomatic disruption, we can judge the religious adaptation to be psychiatrically pathological. (p. 282)

In line with our interpretation, this type of "religious adaptation" falls within the province of psychiatric meanings. Although it may take on distinctively religious language and affect, its pathological origin and solipsistic nature bar it from the religious province of meaning. It is entirely possible to move from one province of meaning to another, but it is not possible to occupy two at the same time in the same way. In short, individuals may move back and forth between the realms of authentic religious consciousness and genuine mental disturbance. Knowing precisely which world someone currently inhabits can be difficult to determine, yet the practical consequences of not knowing can be grave. Saints have been gratuitously slaughtered for their innocent religious practices, and psychotics have merrily committed atrocities in the name of religion.

Herein lies the rationale for a collaborative relationship between religion and psychiatry. The two realms provide parallel vectors of insight and understanding that, while not intersecting, are mutually instructive. "Religion must be concerned with psychological dynamics as these affect and qualify religious functioning" (McCarthy 1990, p. 59). And similarly, "psychology must be concerned with religious and moral issues as psychological factors insofar as they impact on psychological functioning" (McCarthy 1990, p. 59). But, again, the two spheres must remain distinct: "It is not just that psychiatry and religion see things differently. In important respects they see different things" (McCarthy 1990, p. 41). In phenomenological terms, psychiatry and religion are interested in different *meanings* and the manner in which these meanings are constituted by specific activities of the mind. By establishing this point and thus diminishing the potential for some serious confusion, it is now possible to discuss how psychiatry can make appropriate contact with the world of religion, and vice versa.

For example, religious beliefs, objects, and rites are often transferred into the realm of mental disturbance. Although these mental phenomena are not authentically religious, the psychiatrist may rely on religious and theological sources in seeking to understand and treat them. Religious history and theology "can be sources of wisdom in territory that is uncharted by secular society, even if [the] religion that is the source of this wisdom is not one to which an individual might subscribe" (Ahronheim 1994, p. 7). Basic insight into the nature and function of authentic religious consciousness can thus provide important clues regarding the origins of mental disturbance and the potential direction of destructive behaviors associated with it.

Conversely, psychiatric theory and practice can benefit religion, since psychiatric factors can influence the quality of religious functioning. Obsessive scrupulosity or morbid guilt, for example, can find their way into religious practice and ultimately destroy peoples' ability to sustain authentic religious consciousness. Without their explicit knowledge and willing assent, they find themselves shunted into a province of meaning that is inimical to genuine religious experience. Understandably, they easily misconstrue the actual state of affairs, confusing themselves and others, who, regrettably, ascribe their morbid behavior to authentic religion. Confronted with obvious psychiatric symptoms, insightful ministers recognize their limits and make the appropriate referrals, unless they are specially trained in the field of mental health. A skilled psychiatrist can help the confused believer recognize that he or she has exited the field of religious consciousness for alien ranges of experience that are psychiatrically pathological rather than religiously normative.

Religion and Psychiatry: Bioethics as Arbiter of Respect

Although certain absolute distinctions must be acknowledged, it is obvious that the interests of religion and psychiatry intersect significantly. The two spheres provide parallel vectors of insight and guidance as individuals strive to achieve and sustain meaningful, coherent, and morally consistent lives. As in the relationship between any two individuals, communities, or fields of endeavor, ethical concerns arise as competing moral claims come into play when psychiatric practice and religious life meet. The relatively new field of bioethics addresses these ethical quandaries and eases their resolution. It offers a congenial venue for adjudicating the competing, and sometimes contradictory, moral claims of psychiatry and religion. Its methods encourage a thorough assessment of ethical problems and options as they arise at the interface of religion and psychiatry.

Generally understood, bioethics is the systematic identification, analysis, and resolution of ethical problems associated with the biomedical sciences and their application, especially in the practice of medicine. As such, bioethics strives to generate moral insight and [to] offer practical guidance in relevant areas, ranging from the care of individual patients to the development of social policy. In pursuing its goals, bioethics champions a central human question: "What are my duties and obligations to other individuals whose life and well-being may be affected by my actions?" (Callahan 1995, p. 251).

In a pluralistic society like the United States, the duties and obligations of psychiatrists are often conditioned by the religious convictions of the individuals they treat. Discerning right from wrong is not always simple. Bioethics aims at clarifying the moral boundaries of specific cases by elucidating the status of religious belief and pointing to the moral essence of the case under consideration.

For example, in cases of obsessive scrupulosity or morbid guilt that exhibit religious associations, bioethics reminds psychiatrists that they are dealing with pathology, not authentic religion. They are not charged with eliminating childish religious behavior, but rather with freeing the individual from a psychiatric condition that blocks authentic religious consciousness. As for pastors, bioethical analysis alerts them to the existence of a medical rather than a pastoral problem. They have a moral duty to treat it as such. Ethically, the goal here is the restoration of conditions that enable the reemergence of authentic religious consciousness and behavior.

Bioethics also assumes an important mediating role in public policy discussions that seek to balance the respective claims of competent medical practitioners, on the one hand, and the demands of committed religionists, on the other. In the United States, the free-exercise clause of the First Amendment sometimes creates a tension between religious liberty and the practice of medicine. Bioethics brokers the moral interests of both medicine and religion in the development of ethical guidelines governing clinical practice. For example, it promotes a process of moral analysis that supports the choice of an adult Jehovah's Witness not to be transfused and prevents that choice from being disregarded as somehow the result of mental incompetence. Likewise, bioethical analysis may well bolster the arguments of those who claim that their religious beliefs, rather than clinical depression, lead them to actively seek physician-assisted suicide. On the basis of this type of analysis, public policy initiatives will be launched and guidelines developed that seek to honor the integrity of the medical profession while at the same time acknowledging the religious convictions of those who wish to commit suicide.

Although a fully elaborated description of the mediating role of bioethics would require a volume unto itself, the eventual articulation of this role must be guided by one simple precondition: The absolute qualitative distinction between genuine religious consciousness and psychiatrically pathological consciousness must be maintained and acknowledged throughout. Neither psychiatry nor religion has the competence to make authoritative judgments about the internal consistency of the other. Psychiatry is no less ideological than religion, and religion is certainly no less arrogant than psychiatry. Where seemingly irresolvable differences persist, respectful distance must be maintained. Yet, once the essential distinctions discussed in this chapter have been made and the resources of bioethics are employed to mediate the discourse, interaction promises great benefit for both religion and psychiatry.

References

Ahronheim JC, Moreno J, Zuckerman C: Ethics in Clinical Practice. New York, Little, Brown, 1994

Callahan D: Bioethics, in The Encyclopedia of Bioethics, Revised Edition, Vol 1. Edited by Reich WT. New York, Simon & Schuster Macmillan, 1995, pp 247–255

Edie JM: William James and the Phenomenological Thesis of the Primacy of Perception, in Akten des XIV Internationalen Kongresses fur Philosophie, Vol 5. Vienna, Herder, 1969, pp 88–95

Edie JM: William James on the structure of experience. Review of Metaphysics 23:227–238, 1970

Gelder MG: Psychiatry, in The Oxford Companion to Medicine, Vol 2. New York, Oxford University Press, 1986, pp 1147–1158

Husserl E: Experience and Judgment (1939). Translated by Churchill J, Ameriks K. Evanston, IL, Northwestern University Press, 1973

James W: The Principles of Psychology, Vol 2 (1890). New York, Dover, 1950

James W: The Varieties of Religious Experience (1902). London, Collins, 1963

Jones SL: A constructive relationship for religion with the science and profession of psychology. Am Psychol 49:184–199, 1994

Lukoff D, Lu F, Turner R: Toward a more culturally sensitive DSM-IV: psychoreligious and psychospiritual problems. J Nerv Ment Dis 180:673–682, 1992

McCarthy M: A Roman Catholic perspective on psychiatry, in Religious and Ethical Factors in Psychiatric Practice. Edited by Browning DS, Jobe T, Evison IS. Chicago, IL, Nelson-Hall, 1990, pp 41–66

Meissner WW: The phenomenology of religious psychopathology. Bull Menninger Clin 55:281–298, 1991

Post SG: DSM-III-R and religion. Soc Sci Med 35:81–90, 1992

Schutz A: Some leading concepts of phenomenology, in Collected Papers, Vol 1. Edited by Natanson M. The Hague, Netherlands, Martinus Nijhoff, 1941

Smith JE: The Spirit of American Philosophy. New York, Oxford University Press, 1966

Spiegelberg H: The Phenomenological Movement, Vol 1. The Hague, Netherlands, Martinus Nijhoff, 1969

Stephens R: James and Husserl: The Foundations of Meaning. The Hague, Netherlands, Martinus Nijhoff, 1974

Wallace ER: Psychiatry and its nosology: a historical–philosophical overview, in Philosophical Perspectives on Psychiatric Diagnostic Classification. Edited by Sadler JZ, Wiggins OP, Schwartz MA. Baltimore, MD, Johns Hopkins University Press, 1994

Wind JP: Enemies or fellow travelers? religion and psychiatry in the nineteenth century, in Religious and Ethical Factors in Psychiatric Practice. Edited by Browning DS, Jobe T, Evison IS. Chicago, IL, Nelson-Hall, 1990, pp 88–106

eⒼ CHAPTER 9 ⒼꙜ

Religious and Spiritual Issues in Psychiatric Education and Training

Francis G. Lu, M.D.

Many of the developments discussed in this book are relevant to psychiatric education and training. In this chapter I briefly review the historical gap between clinicians and their clients in the area of religious and spiritual beliefs, discuss recent official actions by the American Psychiatric Association (APA) and the Accreditation Council for Graduate Medical Education (ACGME) that establish a sound rationale for inclusion of these topics in coursework for residency training in psychiatry, and present a model curriculum for psychiatric residency training programs.

The Clinician–Patient Gap

In a national survey of psychiatric training programs, Sansome et al. (1990) showed that few residency training programs included didactic coursework on any aspect of religion and that supervision seldom addressed religious issues. The authors stated that "an academic approach to the role of religion in psychiatry warrants consideration" (p. 37). These findings parallel those from a survey of clinical psychologists that documented the very large gap between psychologists' perceptions of the importance of addressing religious and spiritual issues in psychotherapy and the lack of attention to these issues in their clinical supervision and training (Shafranske and Malony 1990). The gap in training for both specialties reflects the gap between the relatively low level of religiosity in mental health professionals and the relatively high level in the general public (Bergin and Payne 1990). M. Scott Peck (1993) characterized this gap for American psychiatry most starkly:

> American psychiatry is, I believe, currently in a predicament. I call it a predicament because its traditional neglect of the issue of spirituality has led to five broad areas of failure: occasional, devastating misdiagnosis; not infrequent mistreatment; an increasingly poor reputation; inadequate research and theory; and a limitation of psychiatrists' own personal development. Taken further, these failures are so destructive to psychiatry that the predicament can properly be called grave. (p. 243)

Recent Encouraging Developments

As a result of the growing recognition that religious/spiritual beliefs and practices are widespread among the general American population and that these beliefs and practices have clinical relevance, the APA and the ACGME began to call for greater sensitivity and better training of clinicians concerning the handling of religious and spiritual issues in the evaluation, assessment, treatment, and care of patients.

In 1990, the APA's Committee on Religion and Psychiatry issued "Guidelines Regarding Possible Conflict Between Psychiatrists' Religious Commitments and Psychiatric Practice," which stated that "psychiatrists should maintain respect for patients' beliefs" (American Psychiatric Association 1990).

The following relevant sections of the APA's "Practice Guidelines for the Psychiatric Evaluation of Adults" (American Psychiatric Association 1995) explicitly characterize religious/spiritual beliefs as essential to the assessment process *(emphasis added)*:

1. "The patient's history of formal education and history of important *cultural and religious influences* on the patient's life are obtained" during the personal history interview (American Psychiatric Association 1995, p. 71).
2. During the patient interview, "the evaluation ought to be performed in a manner that is sensitive to the patient's individuality, identifying issues of development, culture, ethnicity, gender, sexual orientation, familial/genetic patterns, *religious/spiritual beliefs*, social class, and physical and so-

cial environment influencing the patient's symptoms and behavior" (American Psychiatric Association 1995, p. 74).

3. The process of assessment (i.e., diagnosis and case formulation) must include "information specific to the individual patient that goes beyond what is conveyed by the diagnosis. The scope and depth of the formulation vary with the purpose of evaluation. Elements commonly include psychosocial and developmental factors that may have contributed to the present illness; the patient's particular strengths and weaknesses; social resources, and the ability to form and maintain relationships; issues related to culture, ethnicity, gender, sexual orientation, and *religious/spiritual beliefs;* likely precipitating or aggravating factors in the illness; and preferences, and opinions, and biases of the patient relevant to the choice of treatment" (American Psychiatric Association 1995, p. 76).

4. A summary section titled "Consideration of Sociocultural Diversity" states: "The process of psychiatric evaluation must take into consideration and respect the diversity of American subcultures and must be sensitive to the patient's ethnicity and place of birth, gender, social class, sexual orientation, and *religious/spiritual beliefs.* Respectful evaluation involves an empathic, nonjudgmental attitude toward the patient's explanation of illness, concerns, and background. An awareness of one's possible biases or prejudices about patients from different subcultures and an understanding of the limitations of one's knowledge and skills in working with such patients may lead to the identification of situations calling for consultation with a clinician who has expertise concerning a particular subculture. Further, the potential effect of the psychiatrist's sociocultural identity on the attitude and behavior of the patient should be taken into account in the formulation of a diagnostic opinion" (American Psychiatric Association 1995, p. 76).

In the fourth edition of the *Diagnostic and Statistical Manual of Mental Disorders* (DSM-IV; American Psychiatric Association 1994), a nonpathological category, "religious or spiritual problem," was added to the section titled "Other Conditions That May Be a Focus of Clinical Attention" (Lukoff et al. 1992; Turner et al. 1995). Religion is discussed as a possible support for patients in the "Outline for Cultural Formulation" (Appendix I of DSM-IV; also see Lu et al. 1995a), and religious experiences are considered under the "specific culture, age, and gender features" subsections included for each of the major disorders.

The most important development in the effort to incorporate religious/spiritual issues into medical training came in March 1994, when the ACGME distributed the new "Special Requirements for Residency Training in Psychiatry," with which all psychiatry training programs were required to comply beginning January 1, 1995 (American Medical Association 1995). Among the changes to the requirements were two specifically related to religion and spirituality *(emphasis added)*:

1. The didactic curriculum for psychiatric residency training should include a "presentation of the biological, psychological, sociocultural, economic, ethnic, gender, *religious/spiritual*, sexual orientation, and family factors that significantly influence physical and psychological development in infancy, childhood, adolescence, and adulthood."

2. "The residency program should provide its residents with instruction about American culture and subcultures, particularly those found in the patient community associated with the training program. This instruction should include such issues as sex, race, ethnicity, *religion/spirituality*, and sexual orientation."

Finally, publications from the American Counseling Association (Kelly 1995) and the American Psychological Association (Shafranske 1996) point to a growing awareness of the importance of religious/spiritual issues in the training of therapists. Outstanding textbooks on religion and mental health (Schumaker 1992), the religious experience (Hood et al. 1996), transpersonal psychiatry (Scotton et al. 1996), and transpersonal psychotherapy (Boorstein 1996) have also been published. Furthermore, the transpersonal psychiatry and psychology movement endeavored to incorporate religious and spiritual issues into clinical care, training, and research.

A Model Curriculum

The "Special Requirements for Residency Training in Psychiatry" (American Medical Association 1995) establish knowledge, skills, and attitudinal objectives. These objectives, as applied to religious/spiritual experiences, are listed in the following outline (Lu et al. 1995b).

I. Knowledge

The resident should demonstrate competence in the following:

A. Defining the religious/spiritual as encompassing the following phenomenological aspects: experiences/attitudes/practices/beliefs (henceforth to be designated simply "experiences").

B. Understanding the unique impact of religious/spiritual experiences on physical and psychological development in infancy, childhood, adolescence, and adulthood.
C. Understanding the differential diagnostic features of religious/spiritual experiences at both the individual and the organizational level.
D. Understanding the religious/spiritual factors that affect the course and treatment of psychiatric disorders.
E. Understanding the impact of religious/spiritual experiences on the relationship between psychiatrist and patient, including transference and countertransference.
F. Understanding how religious/spiritual issues affect medical ethics as applied to psychiatric practice.
G. Understanding the variety of religious/spiritual experiences and traditions, each with its unique perspective on transpersonal issues.

II. Skills

The resident should demonstrate competence in the following:

A. Interviewing religiously/spiritually committed patients with sensitivity to communication styles, vulnerabilities, and strengths.
B. Listening for religious/spiritual issues in patients' personal narratives, and eliciting accurate and complete histories that reflect an understanding of the importance of these issues in patients' lives.
C. Assessing and diagnosing patients, and formulating treatment plans, in a manner that reflects an understanding of patients' religious/spiritual experiences.
D. Recognizing the features that differentiate normative religious/spiritual experiences from pathological phenomena.
E. Providing appropriate psychotherapeutic interventions that reflect an understanding of patients' religious/spiritual experience.
F. Recognizing and using specific transference and countertransference reactions (negative reactions may indicate unresolved therapist issues in this area).
G. Recognizing possible biases against religious/spiritual issues in the psychiatric literature and understanding their origins.

III. Attitudes

Residents should demonstrate the following in their behavior and demeanor:

A. An awareness of their own religious/spiritual experiences and the impact of these experiences on their identity and worldview.

B. An awareness of their own attitudes toward various religious/spiritual experiences and the possible biases that could influence their assessment and treatment of patients with these experiences.
C. Empathy and respect for patients from a variety of religious/spiritual backgrounds.

A model curriculum on religion and spirituality in clinical practice was recently published (Larson et al. 1997) to assist psychiatry residency training programs in fulfilling the new ACGME requirements. The curriculum is organized into 11 modules that can be integrated into existing training programs. Each module contains the following: 1) objectives (knowledge, skills, attitudes), 2) content, 3) core references, 4) other references, 5) suggested applications, and 6) anticipated problems/barriers.

The first three modules are core modules that present key information:

- Module 1: Religion and Spirituality and Mental Health: An Introductory Overview
- Module 2: Interviewing and Assessing Patients' Religious/Spiritual Practices, Beliefs, and Attitudes
- Module 3: Religion/Spirituality in Human Development: A Tour Through the Life Cycle

Optimally, these three modules would be covered in about six 60- to 90-minute sessions; however, suggestions are provided for prioritization of essential topics for coverage in fewer sessions.

Module 1 provides a brief history of the relationship between psychiatry and religion, presents the research to date linking religion/spirituality with either positive or negative mental health status, and discusses the ethical implications of addressing (or not addressing) religious and spiritual issues in a psychiatric setting. It also examines the various definitions of terms often used in conjunction with religious and spiritual practices and beliefs.

Module 2 provides guidelines for developing a religiously/spiritually sensitive approach to interviewing and assessing patients. Among the topics covered are how to conduct a religious/spiritual history and how to assess the role that religious beliefs play in shaping a patient's personality and worldview. Also covered are the knowledge, skills, and attitudes needed by psychiatrists in order to differentiate between religious/spiritual beliefs that may indicate psychopathology and religious/spiritual beliefs that may potentially benefit or positively influence the patient's mental health. Finally, the module explores transference and countertransference issues.

Module 3 includes a discussion of the influence of religion/spirituality on personality and mental health in childhood and adolescence; religion, spirituality, and sexuality in early adulthood; religion, mental health, and marriage and divorce; religious/spiritual development in late life; and religion/spirituality in death and dying.

The remaining eight modules are accessory modules that present information on additional topics:

- Module 4: The Psychiatry–Medicine Interface: Consultation–Liaison Psychiatry
- Module 5: Collaborating With Clergy in the Assessment and Treatment of the Psychiatric Patient
- Module 6: Religious/Spiritual Issues in the Care and Treatment of Substance Abuse Problems
- Module 7: Religious/Spiritual Issues in the Treatment of Women
- Module 8: Religious/Spiritual Issues in the Treatment of Abused Persons
- Module 9: An Introduction to God Images
- Module 10: An Introduction to Charismatic Religious Experiences
- Module 11: An Introduction to Cults and Their Relationship to Mainstream Religion

These accessory modules may be incorporated into existing didactic courses, case conferences, or clerkship rotations in inpatient, outpatient, and consultation–liaison settings.

The overall attitudinal objectives, which may be the most difficult of the objectives to achieve, might be fulfilled through a variety of learning formats. First, training programs for residents might use an experiential small-group training format similar to that developed by Elaine Pinderhughes (1988) in her work exploring race, ethnicity, and power; her methods could be extended to include religious/spiritual issues. Second, supervisor must be sensitive to religious/spiritual experiences. A small group of faculty with interest and expertise in this area might provide consultation and case-conference discussions, as well as make themselves available as potential supervisors.

Looking Toward the Future

As the population of the United States becomes increasingly multicultural, encompassing people with many different religious and spiritual beliefs, future psychiatric residents will need to gain familiarity with religious/spiritual issues as they are encountered in their practices. Failure to do so risks perpetuation of the problems enumerated by M. Scott Peck (1993; see section titled "The Clinician–Patient Gap" at beginning of chapter), as well as the likelihood of lowered patient satisfaction and poorer patient outcomes.

Furthermore, the rest of the field of medicine has begun to incorporate spirituality into practice and training. For example, in December 1995, a major continuing medical education (CME) course at Harvard titled "Spirituality and Healing in Medicine" drew more than 900 participants. Moreover, in April 1997, the National Institute for Healthcare Research and the Association of American Medical Colleges sponsored a conference called "Spirituality in the Medical School Curriculum"; almost all of the model curricula presented were situated in departments other than psychiatry. If psychiatry continues to neglect this area, it risks the loss of a crucial opportunity to foster an expanded biopsychosocial–spiritual perspective.

In 1998 and 1999, the National Institute for Healthcare Research awarded the John Templeton Foundation Spirituality and Medicine Award to 14 psychiatry residency programs. The awards were funded by the John Templeton Foundation; recipients were selected by a panel of psychiatric educators. The residency programs receiving the awards adapted the model curriculum presented in this chapter for use in their own training approaches.

Teaching methods, including the model curriculum presented here, will need evaluation and ongoing development and refinement. A major remaining challenge is the training of existing faculty in these new perspectives, including the latest empirical studies on religion and psychiatry. Future educational projects might include the following: a casebook to illustrate assessment and treatment planning involving religious/spiritual issues; a guide to films and videotapes useful for training in this area; and the evaluation of additional model curricula projects, not only in the didactic and clerkship portions of psychiatric residency but also in medical student education in psychiatry. Finally, translating and applying the results of ongoing clinical research in this area to specific clinical practice settings will remain an ever-present challenge.

References

American Medical Association: Graduate Medical Education Directory 1995–1996: Program Requirements for Residency Education in Psychiatry. Chicago, IL, American Medical Association, 1995

American Psychiatric Association: Guidelines regarding possible conflict between psychiatrists' religious commitments and psychiatric practice. Am J Psychiatry 147:542, 1990

American Psychiatric Association: Diagnostic and Statistical Manual of Mental Disorders, 4th Edition. Washington, DC, American Psychiatric Association, 1994

American Psychiatric Association: Practice guidelines for the psychiatric evaluation of adults. Am J Psychiatry 152 (11 suppl):64–80, 1995

Bergin AE, Jensen JP: Religiosity of psychotherapists: a national survey. Psychotherapy 27:3–7, 1990

Boorstein S (ed): Transpersonal Psychotherapy, 2nd Edition. Albany, NY, State University of New York Press, 1996

Hood RW, Spilka B, Hunsberger B, et al: The Psychology of Religion: An Empirical Approach, 2nd Edition. New York, Guilford, 1996

Kelly EW: Spirituality and Religion in Counseling and Psychotherapy. Alexandria, VA, American Counseling Association, 1995

Larson DB, Lu FG, Swyers JP: A Model Curriculum for Psychiatry Residency Training Programs: Religion and Spirituality in Clinical Practice, Revised Edition. Rockville, MD, National Institute for Healthcare Research, 1997

Lu FG, Lim RF, Mezzich JE: Issues in the assessment and diagnosis of culturally diverse individuals, in The American Psychiatric Press Annual Review of Psychiatry, Vol 14. Edited by Oldham J, Riba M. Washington, DC, American Psychiatric Press, 1995a, pp 477–510

Lu FG, Bowman E, Juthani N: Psychiatric Training About Religion and Spirituality: Toward a Model Curriculum. Workshop presented at the Mid-Winter Meeting, American Association of Directors of Psychiatric Residency Training, Tucson, AZ, January 14, 1995b

Lukoff D, Lu F, Turner R: Toward a more culturally sensitive DSM-IV: psychoreligious and psychospiritual problems. J Nerv Ment Dis 180:673–682, 1992

Peck MS: Further Along the Road Less Traveled. New York, Simon & Schuster, 1993

Pinderhughes E: Understanding Race, Ethnicity and Power. New York, Free Press, 1988

Sansome RA, Khatain K, Rodenhauser P: The role of religion in psychiatric education: a national survey: Academic Psychiatry 14:34–38, 1990

Schumaker J (ed): Religion and Mental Health. New York, Oxford University Press, 1992

Scotton BW, Chinen A, Battista JR (eds): Textbook of Transpersonal Psychiatry and Psychology. New York, Harper Collins, 1996

Shafranske E (ed): Religion and the Clinical Practice of Psychology. Washington, DC, American Psychological Association, 1996

Shafranske EP, Malony HN: Clinical psychologists' religious and spiritual orientations and their practice of psychotherapy. Psychotherapy 27(1), 1990

Turner RP, Lukoff D, Barnhouse RT, et al: Religious or spiritual problem: a culturally sensitive diagnostic category in the DSM-IV. J Nerv Ment Dis 183:435–444, 1995

⸎ CHAPTER 10 ⸎

Religion and Future Psychiatric Nosology and Treatment

Harold G. Koenig, M.D., M.H.Sc.

In contrast to the separation and conflict that has characterized the relationship between religious and psychiatric professionals during the previous centuries (Zilboorg and Henry 1941), the 21st century holds great promise for increased understanding and collaboration between members of these two disciplines. In this chapter I discuss six major themes: 1) sociodemographic trends affecting the future of religion and psychiatry, 2) implications of these trends for psychiatric diagnosis, 3) implications of these trends for psychiatric treatment, 4) integration of religion into psychiatric practice, 5) integration of religion into psychiatric education, and 6) integration of religion into psychiatric research.

Sociodemographic Trends

The aging of the United States population, the rate of psychiatric disorders in middle-aged and younger adults ("baby boomers"), and dwindling financial resources available for the treatment of psychiatric disorders (Medicare,

Funding for writing this chapter was provided by National Institute of Mental Health Clinical Mental Health Academic Award MH01138.

Medicaid) are trends that will profoundly influence the relationship between religion and psychiatry in the future. The 76-million-member cohort of persons born between 1946 and 1965 has enjoyed a high standard of living, economic prosperity, and a quality of health unknown to previous generations of Americans. Despite this affluence, rates of depression, anxiety, and substance abuse are three to four times more prevalent in this cohort than in persons currently 65 years or older in the United States (Regier et al. 1988). Higher rates of psychiatric disorder in younger cohorts have been confirmed in national surveys (Kessler et al. 1994).

Possible reasons for this trend are too numerous to review here and have been speculated on elsewhere (Klerman and Weissman 1989). As the post–World War II baby-boom generation ages and begins to experience health problems, disability, and reductions in economic prosperity, there is concern that rates of psychiatric disorder may rise even higher. Although people are living longer because of advances in medicine, this is often at the cost of increasing disability and chronic illness. The number of persons with severe disability in this country is rising rapidly, with estimates indicating an increase from 2 million in 1986 to more than 12 million in 2040 (Kunkel and Applebaum 1992) (Figure 10–1). Studies have demonstrated a clear relationship between increasing disability or chronic illness and both depression (Von Korff et al. 1992; Williamson and Schulz 1992) and substance abuse (Moos et al. 1993), suggesting a concomitant rise above current levels in rates of these disorders with time.

Whereas the number of persons with emotional disorders is likely to rise in the years ahead, the financial resources to treat these conditions are declining. Cuts in Medicare and Medicaid are clearly a high priority in the plan to balance the federal budget over the next decade, despite increasing numbers of older persons in need of mental health care; these cuts are predicted to create a mental health crisis as we move into the second quarter of the 21st century (Koenig et al. 1994b). Thus, in the not-too-distant future it is likely that many Americans with emotional disorders, particularly the elderly and impoverished, will be in need of increasingly scarce mental health services (Figure 10–2). Before the development of government social programs, it was often religious bodies that met the health care needs of underprivileged members of society (Braceland and Stock 1963; Stevens 1989); this may also be true in the future. For this reason, as community mental health centers and social service agencies become overwhelmed with demand for services, they will look toward other community groups (e.g., churches) to provide a helping hand. Collaboration among mental health, social service, and religious organizations will be required to respond to the sheer burden of demand.

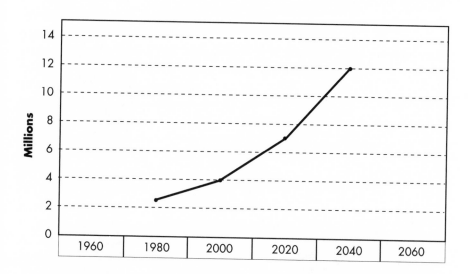

FIGURE 10–1. Current (1980–1990) and projected numbers of severely disabled persons over age 65 years.

Note. Numbers are based on estimates of long-term disability prevalence by Kunkel and Applebaum (1992).

Source. Reprinted from Koenig HG: *Is Religion Good for Your Health?* New York, Haworth, 1997, p. 11. Used with permission.

There is surprisingly little difference in the distribution and severity of psychiatric disorders seen by clergy and those seen by mental health professionals (Larson et al. 1988). There is also considerable receptivity among the American public toward clergy counseling. According to Ross (1993), a Gallup survey reported that 66% of the general population indicated a preference for "a professional counselor who is religious." Likewise, in a survey of Connecticut residents that asked respondents what type of mental health professional they would recommend to a friend (Murstein and Fontaine 1993), 37 cited a psychologist, 32 a psychiatrist, 22 a clergy person, and 21 a social worker.

Thus, the expanding mental health needs of the United States population are likely to compel cooperation among professional groups that provide mental health counseling. For this collaboration to work smoothly and efficiently, members of each profession must put their ideological differences aside, recognize each other's valuable and unique contributions, and be willing to communicate with each other in a collegial manner.

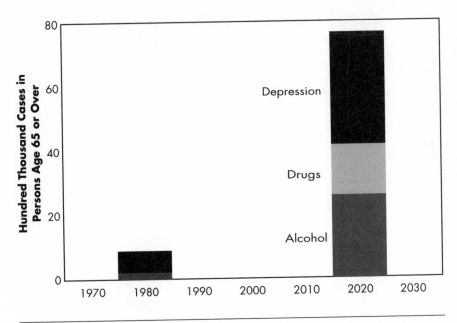

FIGURE 10–2. The mental health-care crisis ahead: current (1980) and projected cases of mental disorders in persons age 65 years or older.
Note. Assuming increasing disability has no effect on cases of mental illness. Projected estimates are based on rates of mental disorder reported by Regier et al. (1988).
Source. Reprinted from Koenig HG: *Is Religion Good for Your Health?* New York, Haworth, 1997, p. 18. Used with permission.

Implications for Psychiatric Diagnosis

Americans are a very religious people. According to a 1995 Gallup poll (Princeton Religion Research Center 1996), more than 95% believe in God and more than 40% attend church weekly. Because religion is so important to many people, it is laden with affect. Consequently, religious themes are often incorporated into delusions and hallucinations of individuals with bipolar disorder, schizophrenia, psychotic depression, or other mental disorders. Furthermore, individuals with personality disorders may have unusual preoccupations with religion or may use it in unhealthy ways. For example, individuals with dependent personality disorder may give "dependence on God" or "waiting on God" as an excuse for inactivity. Those with obsessive-compulsive personality disorder may compulsively pray or engage in other religious rituals, activities that are condoned and even encouraged by some religious groups as a sign of "spirituality." Persons with antisocial personality disorder may use religion to cheat others out of their finances or otherwise manipulate religion to serve their own personal needs. Individuals with borderline personality disorder may funnel rage and anger toward condemning to hell those with beliefs different from their own. Persons with narcissistic personality disorder may set themselves up as religious leaders or spiritual guides in order to attract attention to themselves and their "powers." These are just a few examples of how religion can be used in the service of psychopathology. It is not religion per se, however, that is the problem; rather, religion becomes the vehicle for the expression of psychopathology.

Larson and colleagues (1993) assessed the presentation and interpretation of religion in the area of psychiatric nosology. These authors systematically reviewed the DSM-III-R (American Psychiatric Association 1987) Glossary of Technical Terms (Appendix C) for evidence of bias against religion—and, in particular, for insensitive representations of religion. Of the 45 case examples used in the glossary to illustrate technical terms, 10 (22.2%) had religious content; of these 10, 3 were verbatim patient statements and 7 were descriptions of patient behavior, thinking, or language. The verbatim statements were found in the technical terms "illogical thinking," "incoherence," and "poverty of content and speech"; the descriptions were found in "affect," "catatonic posturing," "delusions of being controlled," "hallucinations, tactile I," "hallucinations, tactile II," "magical thinking," and "delusions." Larson et al. (1993) concluded that religion was overrepresented in case examples of psychopathology. This problem has been largely dealt with in DSM-IV (American Psychiatric Association 1994), which includes a V code for "religious or spiritual problem," indicating greater sensitivity to religious concerns.

Given a better understanding of the role and manifestations of religion in our culture, psychiatrists in the future will become increasingly sensitive to their patients' religious backgrounds and expressions. Psychiatrists will need to seek special knowledge about religious traditions that are unfamiliar to them, particularly Fundamentalist Christianity, New Age spirituality, Buddhism, Hinduism, and Islam, as well as seek information about the larger religious cults. Such knowledge will help them to better identify the fine line between healthy religious expression and psychopathology. In many cases, mental health professionals will need to seek input from clergy familiar with the religious beliefs, practices, and experiences of members of these groups.

Implications for Psychiatric Treatment

A greater understanding of the meaning and importance of religion in the lives of patients will affect the design of treatment plans by prompting psychiatrists to consider cultural factors and belief systems that may influence patients' acceptance of—and thus, their compliance with—these treatments. Religious systems of healing, however, may not always blend easily with psychiatric therapies. For example, patients may experience conflict when attempting to decide whether to put their trust and faith in God for healing, or to put it in their therapist, medication, or electroconvulsive therapy; indeed, distressing guilt may be experienced when they seek assistance from mental health professionals because of these conflicting feelings. Unless such issues are addressed by therapists, they may lead to noncompliance. There are movements within some areas of Fundamentalist Christianity and other religious groups (e.g., Christian Scientists) that vehemently oppose psychotherapy in particular, because it competes with the religious system of healing (Bobgan and Bobgan 1989). Furthermore, the specific attitudes and behaviors encouraged during psychotherapy (particularly cognitive-behavioral therapy) may conflict with or run counter to the laws and teachings of religious groups. For example, emphasis in secular psychotherapy on getting personal needs met and on self-fulfillment may run counter to religious teachings that encourage loving and serving others, suffering, and self-sacrifice.

The use of psychotropic medications may also conflict with the belief systems of certain religious groups, for the same reason that such use is resisted by some psychotherapists. For example, we now possess in our armamentarium drugs that can effectively relieve, if not eliminate, anxiety. This reduction in anxiety may reduce the patient's desire for change and growth. There is an optimum level of anxiety necessary to motivate individuals to continue the hard work involved in changing thinking and/or behavior, as required in both psychotherapy and spiritual practice. Thus, the use of medication that reduces or eliminates anxiety may reduce motivation and drive toward personal and spiritual growth, and thus may be opposed by religious groups. Again, unless the psychiatrist is aware of this issue and addresses it in therapy, it may undermine even the best of therapeutic plans. A two-pronged approach—education of clergy on the uses of psychotropic medication and careful titration of doses to eliminate dysfunctional anxiety and preserve functional anxiety—may be necessary to achieve optimal results.

In a study of more than 850 Protestant baby boomers surveyed in the National Institute of Mental Health Epidemiologic Catchment Area program, findings showed that members of Pentecostal denominations had higher rates of psychiatric disorder than did members of other religious groups; rates were especially high among members who attended church *infrequently*, a group that also seldom (if ever) sought help from mental health professionals (no one in this group had made an outpatient mental health visit within the previous 6 months) (Koenig et al. 1994a). These findings suggest a need for collaboration between Pentecostal churches and mental health providers to reach out to church members with mental health problems who may not be receiving help from either group.

Finally, as noted earlier, normative religious experience (especially that which is unfamiliar to the therapist) may be confused with symptoms of psychopathology. Our increasing knowledge about religious experience and phenomena may help us determine which symptoms to treat and which symptoms to observe and support. The following case description illustrates this principle.

Tom, a 22-year-old college student, was brought by family members to see a psychiatrist because he had returned home one night after a religious revival claiming that God had spoken to him and called him to leave school and become a Christian missionary in Africa. Tom, who had previously shown little interest in religion, reported that during the revival he had experienced a sudden, profound sense of peace, during which his senses became vividly clear and he heard a voice (which he perceived as God) telling him to give up all his possessions and preach the Gospel in Africa. This was followed by the insight that all of the experiences in his life prior to that time had prepared him for this calling. Further questioning by the psychiatrist of Tom and his family revealed that he had never had any types of hallucinations before, that his behavior prior to that night and performance in school had been normal, and that he had not taken any drugs or hallucinogens recently. The psychiatrist decided to monitor the patient on a weekly and then monthly basis but to refrain from recommending further treatment for the time being. There was no progression in his symptoms (hearing the voice), although his sense of calling remained. After several months, Tom left school and joined a missionary group in Africa. Follow-up several years later found him content and fulfilled, pursuing a successful ministry in Tanzania.

In this case, the psychiatrist's knowledge about the religious background of the patient and his careful evaluation and follow-up to observe for symptom progression and effect on functioning were the keys to successful management.

Integration of Religion Into Psychiatric Practice

Rather than competing with one another over delivery of mental health care, psychiatrists and clergy should try to complement and work with one another. They must learn to recognize the limits and boundaries of their respective professions and be aware of each other's strengths and weaknesses. For example, psychiatrists have expertise in the diagnosis of mental disorders and possess the specific therapeutic skills needed to treat some of these disorders. The diagnosis and treatment of bipolar disorder, major depressive disorder, panic disorder, schizophrenia, delusional disorder, dementia and other cognitive disorders, and the more severe personality and addictive disorders are done by psychiatrists because of their special training in and experience with patients who have these conditions. On the other hand, many of the minor depressions, milder forms of major depression, mild to moderate anxiety, and minor adjustment and coping difficulties that plague a much larger proportion of the population can be handled quite well in the pastoral care setting.

Initial screening for the more severe psychiatric disorders should optimally occur at the religious community level to ensure early recognition and timely referral to psychiatric professionals. After diagnosis and treatment have been initiated by mental health professionals, clergy could assist in the follow-up of such patients by supporting the treatment plan, carefully monitoring for compliance, and observing the patient for disease exacerbations or flare-ups. Psychiatrists, in turn, could educate clergy about the more severe psychiatric disorders to assist them in recognizing and managing these conditions; furthermore, psychiatrists could provide guidelines to help clergy determine when clients with milder psychiatric conditions should be referred for more specialized treatments. Thus, close collaboration among psychiatrists, patients, families, clergy, and the faith community (with confidentiality preserved, of course) holds the best hope for meeting mental health care needs in a timely, coordinated, and cost-efficient manner.

Because meeting psychological needs and meeting spiritual needs are overlapping concerns of both psychiatrists and clergy, the boundaries between the two professional realms of concern must necessarily be blurred to some extent. There may be times when the psychiatrist must minister to spiritual needs of patients because the timing for intervention requires this. At other times, the clergy or pastoral counselor may need to address purely psychological concerns, again because the timing of intervention requires this. The focus throughout, however, remains on the patient's needs and on a healthy recognition of each professional's strengths and weaknesses. To work successfully, this collaboration will require clear communication between religious and psychiatric professionals—much clearer (and with greater mutual respect) than now exists between these two groups.

How and when might psychiatrists address the spiritual concerns of patients so that they do not overstep their boundaries of expertise? Just as pastoral counselors must be aware of their patients' previous psychiatric histories and the quality of their interpersonal relationships, psychiatrists must know something about the religious histories of patients, including information about prior positive and negative experiences with religion. Thus, taking a religious history should be a routine part of the initial evaluation of all psychiatric patients. Furthermore, in patients for whom religion is important, psychiatrists must consider and include this fact in their treatment plans. Propst and colleagues (1992) have demonstrated the usefulness and effectiveness of integrating religion into psychotherapy with religious patients. Their study, which included both religious and nonreligious therapists, showed that use of a religious version of cognitive-behavioral therapy (CBT) with religious patients resulted in quicker resolution of depressive symptoms than did use of traditional CBT. In fact, the results achieved by the nonreligious therapists were at least as good as, if not better than, the results achieved by the religious therapists. This finding demonstrates that any therapist—regardless of his or her personal religious background—can effectively treat religious patients when religion is used in therapy.

It is likely, then, that in the future, psychiatrists will make use of the religious beliefs of their patients to help them achieve more rapid results. If psychiatrists choose to do this, however, they must be acutely aware of boundary issues and of sticky countertransference problems that can arise. Such areas become more of a problem when the religious backgrounds of the therapist and patient differ. Because of the zeal with which personal religious beliefs and commitments are typically held, therapists must be cautious not to impose their own religious views and philosophies onto troubled, vulnerable patients. The therapeutic encounter is no place for debating the truth or falsehood of religious doctrines or manipulating patients' attitudes or behaviors to conform with therapists' needs. Moshe Spero (1981) has provided detailed guidelines for addressing problems with transference and countertransference that therapists may face when using religion in psychotherapy.

Especially controversial are religious interventions initiated by psychiatrists, such as prayer or use of religious scriptures to direct patients' attitudes or behaviors. Such interventions test the boundaries between psychiatric and religious areas of expertise. In a general medical setting, the use of prayer is by no means rare; surveys demonstrate that one-third of family physicians have prayed with their patients (Koenig et al. 1989) and that the majority of patients are receptive to such interventions (King and Bushwick 1994; Koenig et al. 1988). The issue of praying with patients, however, is more delicate in psychiatry than in primary care. This is because psychiatrists often deal with mentally unstable individuals with unclear boundaries, who may perceive and respond to religious interventions in unpredictable ways. Nevertheless, prayer may be useful in carefully selected situations (e.g., times of acute stress precipitated by real-life events, where religious professionals may not be readily available) or with religious patients with adequate ego functioning who have given explicit, uncoerced permission to the therapist for such activity (see Koenig et al. 1996 for a more complete discussion of this issue).

Thus, the future of psychiatry and religion as it relates to psychiatric practice will involve increased collaboration and communication between psychiatrists and clergy, and a greater freedom by psychiatrists to address religious issues and (to a more limited extent) utilize the religious resources of patients in therapy.

Integration of Religion Into Psychiatric Education

The importance of educating psychiatrists early in their training to be sensitive to the religious backgrounds, experiences, and conflicts of their patients and to recognize the effects that religion can have on mental health (either positive or negative) was discussed in Chapter 9 of this volume. Some of these points I will repeat and emphasize here, as we look toward the future.

In order to address and understand religious issues in patients, psychiatrists must have a working knowledge of the main religious traditions represented in the United States population. Of the 91% of Americans who claim a religious preference, 93% are Christian, 2% are Jewish, and the remaining 5% are affiliated with Islamic, Hindu, Buddhist, and other religious groups; these percentages have remained relatively stable over the past 50 years (Princeton Religion Research Center 1985) and are unlikely to change much in the near future. Among Christians, approximately two-thirds are Protestants and one-third are Catholics. Among Protestants, 35% are Baptist; 16%, Methodist; 12%, Lutheran; 5%, Episcopalian; 4%, Presbyterian; 4%, United Church of Christ; 4%, Christian Church; and 10%, other Protestants (including Pentecostals, Jehovah's Witnesses, Seventh-Day Adventists, and Mormons). Rather than focus their attention on small religious groups or cults, psychiatrists should be familiar with the beliefs, teachings, and rituals of the major religious groups in America, especially Christian denominations and Judaism, major Eastern religious traditions (Buddhism, Hinduism, and Islam), and New Age spirituality, particularly their teachings on health.

Early in their training, psychiatrists should be exposed to clergy working as part of the health care team (inpatient and outpatient). Chaplains may be included as a regular part of the consultation–liaison team seeing medical inpatients and/or the psychiatric inpatient team caring for persons with severe mental illness. Exposure early in training will help psychiatrists realize the important contributions that clergy can make to the understanding of patients and the development of effective treatment plans. Training in outpatient psychiatry should include experience communicating with community clergy and pastors about patients, taking referrals from clergy, and learning to educate clergy about mental health issues in a nonarrogant and tactful manner.

Finally, psychiatrists must be made aware of the positive as well as the potentially negative effects of religion on mental health. Although religion has for years been considered by mental health professionals to have a largely negative influence on mental health (Ellis 1980; Freud 1927), their case may have been overstated. In fact, more recent research has demonstrated that devout personal religiousness and active involvement in a religious faith community may have distinctly beneficial effects on both physical and mental health (Koenig and Futterman 1995; Koenig et al. 1992; Levin and Schiller 1987; Levin et al. 1995; Matthews and Larson 1993–1995; Williams et al. 1991). Most psychiatrists are not aware of these findings and, because of the prevailing negative attitude toward religion in the field, may have only a one-sided picture of religion's mental health effects. The exposure of psychiatric residents to this research early in training may help to dispel some of the negative biases so prevalent today. Indeed, in March 1994, the Accreditation Council for Graduate Medical Education distributed new "Special Requirements for Residency Training in Psychiatry," which state that didactic curricula must include the presentation of "religious/spiritual" factors that significantly influence physical and psychological development.

With greater freedom to explore and make use of patients' religious beliefs in therapy, psychiatrists will require training to help them recognize boundaries and the effects on the therapeutic alliance of introducing religion (in terms of exacerbating transference and countertransference issues, as discussed previously).

Integration of Religion Into Psychiatric Research

Studies have shown that many, if not most, Americans use religion to help them to cope, particularly during times of acute stress (Koenig 1995). Further studies are necessary to compare the effects of religious coping with those of nonreligious coping behaviors (e.g., distracting activities, support from family) on mental health and emotional well-being. Although recent research has emphasized the health-promoting effects of devout religiousness, relatively few investigations have attempted to identify the specific elements of religious coping that are beneficial—or to isolate types of religious coping that are detrimental to health, as has been suggested by some earlier investigators (Rokeach 1960; Salzman 1953; Sanua 1969). Certain religious groups may exert a control over their members that is almost hypnotic in its extent, so that members' free will is jeopardized. Likewise, rigid, narrow thinking and intolerance of other opinions or views may foster maladaptive, inflexible coping practices. On the other hand, groups emphasizing religious teachings that promote compassion, forgiveness, altruism, positive thinking, and healthy behaviors may foster adaptive coping practices. These aspects of religious belief and practice must be subjected to careful systematic study.

With a few exceptions (Blazer and Palmore 1976; Idler and Kasl 1992; Koenig et al. 1992; Markides et al. 1987), most research examining the relationship between religiousness and mental health has been cross-sectional. Although cross-sectional studies provide information about *association*, they do not elucidate causality or direction of effect. Longitudinal, prospective studies or clinical trials are necessary to yield information about the time sequence of events. If a cross-sectional study shows that people who are more religious are more likely to have mental illness, this sheds little light on religion's effects on mental health; such a finding might simply reflect a turning to religion (as a source of comfort or as a coping behavior) on the part of emotionally disturbed people (just as one might find a positive association between being in a psychiatrist's office and being emotionally disturbed). Likewise, the cross-sectional finding that less-religious people are more depressed than are religious people might simply reflect the effect of depression on religiousness; in other words, as people become more depressed, they may simply lose interest in religion or withdraw from participation in the religious community. An inverse association between religiousness and depression, then, might reflect an effect of depression on religiousness but say nothing about the effectiveness of religion in helping to relieve or prevent depression.

For these reasons, it is imperative that future studies examining the religion–mental health relationship employ longitudinal study designs. Prospective studies will allow us to answer the following questions. Do persons who are more religiously committed at time 1 and who then undergo some type of stress have better mental health at time 2 (after the stress) than those who are not religious at time 1? Alternatively, among those who are depressed or emotionally ill, do persons who turn to religion as a coping behavior recover more quickly than people who cope in nonreligious ways? These are testable hypotheses that require prospective, longitudinal study designs. Such studies are usually expensive and time-consuming, and few funding agencies are willing to provide the type of support necessary to conduct and complete such research. One solution is to include measures of religiousness in longitudinal studies that seek to answer other questions about mental health outcomes or service use; unfortunately, because of space limitations, this strategy often restricts the detail about religious belief and behavior that can be assessed. Nevertheless, until funds become more available to study the religion–mental health connection, piggybacking religious variables onto research questionnaires designed for other purposes seems the most feasible approach.

Other important questions requiring investigation include the following:

1. What is the association between religious affiliation and distribution of psychiatric disorders in the general population? Among religious groups with higher rates of psychiatric disorders, did disorders precede or follow members' affiliation with these groups, and how does severity of illness change over time?
2. What is the association between religious affiliation and use of mental health services by the general population? How does individual religious belief and practice affect use of mental health services?
3. What religious beliefs and practices are most common among persons in good mental health? More important, what religious beliefs and practices are most common among persons in good mental health despite having undergone major developmental traumas, adult life stresses, or severe physical illnesses?
4. How might the healthy components of religion be integrated into psychotherapy with religious patients, and how might religion best be used as a resource and tool in therapy? More randomized clinical trials are needed to examine the effects of religious interventions (e.g., prayer, scripture reading, healing services) in persons with depression or anxiety.
5. How might community mental health agencies, social services, and religious organizations best work together? Pilot projects are needed to test

such collaborative ventures in order to identify and solve the problems that will inevitably arise.

6. What is the best way to educate psychiatric professionals about the contributions that clergy can make to patient care? What is the best way to educate clergy about the role of psychiatrists? Again, pilot projects are needed to assess different approaches.

Conclusions

In the future, we will see closer working relationships develop between psychiatric and religious professionals. The ever-increasing mental health needs of the American people, together with declines or limitations in funding for mental health care, will literally force such collaboration. Mental health professionals must educate clergy about the signs, symptoms, and treatment of psychiatric disorders so that they can recognize these disorders in their congregations. Clergy, on the other hand, must educate mental health professionals about religious beliefs, attitudes, and practices that affect people's lives and health care decisions. Chaplains or other religious professionals must be integrated into health teams that provide care for mentally ill patients in hospital and outpatient settings. Finally, mental health professionals must be willing to reach out to religious organizations, showing themselves friendly and willing to cooperate, even to the point of participating on church boards where possible. Although these notions may seem revolutionary in comparison with past practices, they hold our best chance of effectively and efficiently meeting the mental health needs of Americans for decades to come.

References

Accreditation Council for Graduate Medical Education: Special Requirements for Residency Training in Psychiatry. Chicago, IL, Accreditation Council for Graduate Medical Education, March 1994

American Psychiatric Association: Diagnostic and Statistical Manual of Mental Disorders, 3rd Edition, Revised. Washington, DC, American Psychiatric Association, 1987

American Psychiatric Association: Diagnostic and Statistical Manual of Mental Disorders, 4th Edition. Washington, DC, American Psychiatric Association, 1994

Blazer DG, Palmore E: Religion and aging in a longitudinal panel. Gerontologist 16:82–85, 1976

Bobgan M, Bobgan D: Prophets of Psychoheresy I. Santa Barbara, CA, EastGate Publishers, 1989

Braceland FJ, Stock M: Modern Psychiatry. Garden City, NY, Doubleday, 1963, p 29

Ellis A: Psychotherapy and atheistic values: a response to A. E. Bergin's "Psychotherapy and Religious Values." J Consult Clin Psychol 48:635–639, 1980

Freud S: The future of an illusion (1927), in The Standard Edition of the Complete Psychological Works of Sigmund Freud, Vol 21. Translated and edited by Strachey J. London, Hogarth, 1961, pp 1–56

Idler EL, Kasl SV: Religion, disability, depression, and the timing of death. Am J Sociol 97:1052–1079, 1992

Kessler RC, McGonagle KA, Zhao S, et al: Lifetime and 12-month prevalence of DSM-III-R psychiatric disorders in the United States. Arch Gen Psychiatry 51:8–19, 1994

King DE, Bushwick B: Beliefs and attitudes of hospital inpatients about faith healing and prayer. J Fam Pract 39:349–352, 1994

Klerman GL, Weissman MM: Increasing rates of depression. JAMA 261:2229–2235, 1989

Koenig HG: Faith and spirituality as a means of coping with stress. Theology News and Notes 42:6–8, 22, 1995

Koenig HG: Is Religion Good for Your Health? New York, Haworth, 1997

Koenig HG, Futterman A: Religion and health outcomes: a review and synthesis of the literature (background paper), in Proceedings of Conference on Methodological Approaches to the Study of Religion, Aging, and Health (March 16–17, 1995; sponsored by the National Institute on Aging and the Fetzer Institute). Kallamazoo, MI, Fetzer Institute, 1995

Koenig HG, Smiley M, Gonzales JP: Religion, Health and Aging. Westport, CT, Greenwood, 1988

Koenig HG, Bearon L, Dayringer R: Physician perspectives on the role of religion in the physician–older patient relationship. J Fam Pract 28:441–448, 1989

Koenig HG, Cohen HJ, Blazer DG, et al: Religious coping and depression in elderly hospitalized medically ill men. Am J Psychiatry 149:1693–1700, 1992

Koenig HG, George LK, Meador KG, et al: Religious affiliation and psychiatric disorder among Protestant baby boomers. Hospital and Community Psychiatry 45:586–596, 1994a

Koenig HG, George LK, Schneider R: Mental health care for older adults in the year 2020: a dangerous and avoided topic. Gerontologist 34:674–679, 1994b

Koenig HG, Larson DB, Matthews D: Religion and psychotherapy with older adults. Journal of Geriatric Psychiatry 29:155–184, 1996

Kunkel SR, Applebaum RA: Estimating the prevalence of long-term disability for an aging society. J Gerontol 47:S253–S260, 1992

Larson DB, Hohmann AA, Kessler LG, et al: The couch and the cloth: the need for linkage. Hospital and Community Psychiatry 39:1064–1069, 1988

Larson DB, Thielman SB, Greenwold MA, et al: Religious content in the DSM-III-R glossary of technical terms. Am J Psychiatry 150:1884–1885, 1993

Levin JS, Schiller PL: Is there a religious factor in health? Journal of Religion and Health 26:9–36, 1987

Levin JS, Chatters LM, Taylor RJ: Religious effects on health status and life satisfaction among Black Americans. J Gerontol B Psychol Sci Soc Sci 50:S154–S163, 1995

Markides KS, Levin JS, Ray LA: Religion, aging, and life satisfaction: an eight-year three-wave longitudinal study. Gerontologist 27:660–665, 1987

Matthews DA, Larson DB: The Faith Factor: An Annotated Bibliography of Clinical Research on Spiritual Subjects (Vols I–III). Rockville, MD, National Institute for Healthcare Research, 1993–1995

Moos RH, Mertens JR, Brennan PL: Patterns of diagnosis and treatment among late-middle-aged and older substance abuse patients. J Stud Alcohol 54:479–487, 1993

Murstein BI, Fontaine PA: The public's knowledge about psychologists and other mental health professionals. Am Psychol 48:839–845, 1993

Princeton Religion Research Center: Religion in America—50 Years: 1935–1985 (Gallup Report No. 236). Princeton, NJ, Princeton Religion Research Center, 1985

Princeton Religion Research Center: Will the Vitality of the Church Be the Surprise of the 21st Century? (Gallup Poll). Princeton, NJ, Princeton Religion Research Center, 1996

Propst LR, Ostrom R, Watkins P, et al: Comparative efficacy of religious and nonreligious cognitive-behavioral therapy for the treatment of clinical depression in religious individuals. J Consult Clin Psychol 60:94–103, 1992

Regier DA, Boyd JH, Burke JD, et al: One-month prevalence of mental disorders in the United States: based on five Epidemiologic Catchment Area sites. Arch Gen Psychiatry 45:977–986, 1988

Rokeach M: The Open and Closed Mind. New York, Basic Books, 1960

Ross RJ: Future of pastoral counseling: legal and financial concerns, in The Future of Pastoral Counseling: Whom, How and For What Do We Train? Edited by McHolland J. Fairfax, VA, American Association of Pastoral Counselors, 1993, p 115

Salzman L: The psychology of religious ideological conversion. Psychiatry 16:177–187, 1953

Sanua VD: Religion, mental health, and personality. Am J Psychiatry 125:1203–1213, 1969

Spero MH: Countertransference in religious therapists of religious patients. Am J Psychother 35:565–575, 1981

Stevens R: In Sickness and in Wealth: American Hospitals in the 20th Century. New York, Basic Books, 1989

Von Korff M, Ormel J, Katon W, et al: Disability and depression among high utilizers of health care. Arch Gen Psychiatry 49:91–100, 1992

Williams DR, Larson DB, Buckler RE, et al: Religion and psychological distress in a community sample. Soc Sci Med 32:1257–1262, 1991

Williamson GM, Schulz R: Pain, activity restriction, and symptoms of depression among community-residing elderly adults. J Gerontol 47:P367–P372, 1992

Zilboorg G, Henry GW: A History of Medical Psychology. New York, WW Norton, 1941

Index

*Page numbers printed in **boldface** type refer to tables or figures.*